WHO Technical Report Series

The Selection and Use of Essential Medicines

Report of the WHO Expert Committee, 2011
(including the 17th WHO Model List of Essential Medicines
and the 3rd WHO Model List of Essential Medicines for Children)

This report contains the collective views of an international group of experts and does not necessarily represent the decisions or the stated policy of the World Health Organization

World Health Organization

WHO Library Cataloguing-in-Publication Data:

The selection and use of essential medicines: report of the WHO Expert Committee, March 2011 (including the 17th WHO model list of essential medicines and the 3rd WHO model list of essential medicines for children).

(WHO technical report series ; no. 965)

1. Essential drugs - administration and dosage. 2. Drug information services. 3. Drug utilization. 4. Child. I. World Health Organization. II. Series.

ISBN 978 92 4 120965 6 (NLM classification: QV 55)
ISSN 0512-3054

Printed in Italy

Contents

Executive summary

The 18th Meeting of the WHO Expert Committee on the Selection and Use of Essential Medicines took place in Accra, Ghana on 21–25 March 2011. This was the first meeting of the Committee held outside of Geneva. The purpose of the meeting was to review and update the WHO Model List of Essential Medicines (EML) as well as the WHO Model List of Essential Medicines for Children (EMLc). The Expert Committee Members and Temporary Advisers who participated in the meeting are listed in the report, together with their declarations of interest.

In accordance with its approved procedures (http://apps.who.int/gb/archive/pdf_files/EB109/eeb1098.pdf) the Expert Committee evaluated the scientific evidence on the comparative effectiveness, safety and cost–effectiveness of medicines to update the WHO Model List of Essential Medicines and the Model List of Essential Medicines for Children. The Expert Committee:

- approved the addition of 16 new medicines to the EML;
- approved the deletion of 13 medicines from the EML;
- approved new indications for 4 medicines already listed on the EML;
- approved the addition of a new dosage form or strength for 4 medicines already on the EML;
- rejected 9 applications for the addition of a medicine to EML;
- approved the addition of 16 new medicines to the EMLc;
- approved the deletion of 15 medicines from the EMLc;
- rejected 3 applications for the addition of a new medicine to the EMLc.

Some of the main recommendations made, in order of their appearance on the Model List, were:

- Section 6: addition of artesunate + amodiaquine combination tablet for the treatment of malaria in adults and children, in line with current WHO treatment guidelines. In making its decision, the 2011 Committee reviewed the latest clinical evidence and the information about licensing in several countries of the fixed-dose combination tablet. The Committee noted, however, that appropriate doses of both medicines can also be achieved using combinations of the mono-component products, including co-blistered presentations.
- Section 10: addition of tranexamic acid injection for the treatment of adult patients with trauma and significant risk of ongoing haemorrhage. On the basis of the results of a very large trial of the

use of tranexamic acid specifically for trauma patients — including those who have been in road traffic accidents, the Committee concluded that there is sufficient evidence to support the proposal that listing tranexamic acid may contribute to a reduction in this cause of death.

- Section 18.5: addition of glucagon injection, 1 mg/ml to treat acute severe hypoglycaemia in patients with diabetes, to support efforts in many countries to ensure appropriate treatment of the increasing number of patients with diabetes. The Committee also recommended that careful attention be paid to the cost of procuring glucagon and noted that based on the experience with other high-cost medicines, such as the antiretrovirals, inclusion in the EML may help reduce prices.
- Section 22.1: addition of misoprostol tablet, 200 micrograms for the prevention of postpartum haemorrhage, where oxytocin is not available or cannot be safely used. WHO guidelines currently recommend that *in situations where there is no other treatment available*, misoprostol can be used to prevent and treat postpartum haemorrhage due to uterine atony. New evidence submitted to the Committee shows that misoprostol can be safely administered to women to *prevent* postpartum haemorrhage by traditional birth attendants or assistants trained to use the product at home deliveries. Misoprostol should *not*, however, be used *to treat* haemorrhage unless there is no other option available (see below). Moreover, if it is available, oxytocin is recommended as it is more effective and cheaper.

Other medicines that were added to the Model List are: isoflurane, propofol, midazolam, clarithromycin, miltefosine, paclitaxel and docetaxel, bisoprolol, terbinafine cream/ointment, mupirocin cream/ointment, and atracurium.

The Expert Committee did not approve the following proposals for addition of medicines on the basis of the evidence submitted: ether, gatifloxacin, a fixed-dose combination of isoniazid + pyridoxine + sulfamethoxazole + trimethoprim (because there is no marketed product), etravirine, darunavir, raltegravir, dihydroartemisinin + piperaquine, pyronaridine + artesunate, loperamide and misoprostol tablet for treatment of postpartum haemorrhage.

The Expert Committee also assessed a review of the comparative effectiveness and cost–effectiveness of analogue insulins compared to recombinant human insulin. The products considered were: insulin glargine, insulin detemir, insulin aspart, insulin lispro, and insulin glulisine. The Committee noted that while many of the comparative trials find a statistically significant difference between analogue insulins and standard recombinant human insulin for some effects on blood glucose measurements, there is no evidence of a clinically significant difference in most outcomes. The Committee concluded that insulin analogues currently offer no significant clinical advantage over recombinant human insulin and there is still concern about possible long-term adverse effects.

A summary of reasons for all changes to the List is in Section 1 of the report. All applications and documents considered by the Committee will remain available on the web site for the meeting at: http://www.who.int/selection_medicines/committees/expert/18/en/index.html.

List of participants of the 18th Expert Committee on the Selection and Use of Essential Medicines

Members:

Professor Hany Abdel-Aleem, Department of Obstetrics and Gynecology, Women Health Centre, Assiut University Hospital, Assiut, Egypt

Dr Lisa A Bero, Professor, University of California, San Francisco, USA

Professor Abdol Majid Cheraghali, Iranian Blood Transfusion Organization, Hemmat Highway, Tehran, Islamic Republic of Iran

Professor Noël Cranswick, Clinical Pharmacologist, Royal Children's Hospital, Parkville, Victoria, Australia

Professor Rohini Fernandopulle, Senior Lecturer, Department of Pharmacology, Faculty of Medicine, University of Colombo, Colombo, Sri Lanka

Mr Andy Gray, Department of Therapeutics and Medicines Management, Nelson R. Mandela School of Medicine, University of KwaZulu-Natal, Congella, South Africa

Dr Kalle Hoppu, Director, Poison Information Centre, Helsinki University Central Hospital, Helsinki, Finland

Dr Gregory L Kearns, Professor of Pediatrics and Pharmacology, University of Missouri Kansas City (UMKC), Kansas City, USA (by telephone)

Professor David Ofori-Adjei, Professor of Tropical Clinical Pharmacology, Professor of Medicine & Therapeutics, Noguchi Memorial Institute for Medical Research, University of Ghana, Accra, Ghana

Dr Lenita Wannmacher, former Professor of Clinical Pharmacology, Faculty of Medicine, Federal University of Rio Grande do Sul, Brazil and Consultant and Senior Lecturer on Selection and Rational Use of Medicines for the Brazilian Ministry of Health and the National Health Vigilance Agency, Porto Alegre, Brazil

Professor Anita Zaidi, Associate Professor, Department of Pediatrics and Microbiology, Aga Khan University, Karachi, Pakistan

Temporary Advisers:

Dr Agnès Saint Raymond, European Medicines Agency, London, United Kingdom

Professor Jennifer Welbeck, Department of Child Health, University of Ghana Medical School, Korle Bu Teaching Hospital, Accra, Ghana

Agencies:

UNICEF

Mr Henrik Nielsen, Technical Specialist, Essential Medicines and Nutrition Centre, UNICEF Supply Division, The United Nations Children's Fund (UNICEF), Copenhagen, Denmark

UNFPA

Dr Kabir U Ahmed, Technical Adviser, Commodity Security Branch, Technical Division, United Nations Population Fund (UNFPA), New York, USA

Region:

Dr Analia Porrás, Advisor, Medicines and Technology, HSS/MT (Region of the Americas/ Pan American Health Organization)

WHO Country Office/Ghana:

Dr Daniel Kertesz, WHO Representative to Ghana

Mrs Edith Andrews Annan, Country Adviser-Essential Medicines, World Health Organization, Accra, Ghana

WHO HQ/Secretariat:

Dr Clive Ondari, Coordinator, MAR
Dr Suzanne Hill, Secretary of the Expert Committee, MAR
Dr Anna Ridge, MAR
Ms Monique Renevier, MAR

Declaration of interests of Members of the 18th Expert Committee on the Selection and Use of Essential Medicines

Members reported the following interests:

Professor Noël Cranswick reported receiving honoraria and travel expenses (including economy airfares) from GlaxoSmithKline to produce guidelines and present to multiple audiences on the use of antipyretic medicines in fever and to act as a consultant on the use of paracetamol in children. He was therefore asked to contribute to the discussions but not to any recommendations related to the use of ibuprofen in children.

Mr Andy Gray reported having accepted travel support from Aspen Pharmacare and Fresenius Kabi to attend continuing education events as a guest speaker, and receiving research support grants from Gilead Sciences and various donors of antiretroviral medicines used in AIDS Clinical Trials Group (ACTG) and International Maternal Pediatric Adolescent AIDS Clinical Trials Network (IMPAACT) trials. He reported being a member of the Scheduling and Naming Expert Committee of the South African Medicines Control Council; being a past director of a government funding agency for biotechnology and a non-executive director of a non-profit-making company engaged in the development and implementation of information technology-based health care solutions for the developing world. He was therefore asked not to contribute to recommendations on antiretrovirals.

Dr Kalle Hoppu reported receiving lecture fees from Oy Swedish Orphan AB, Norit Pharmaceuticals, and a consultancy fee from Oy Leiras Finland AB for providing a written clinical expert opinion for a regulatory submission.

Dr Gregory L Kearns reported receiving research grants from the National Institute of Health, the Pediatric Trials Network, MPEX Pharmaceuticals, and Johnson & Johnson; he also declared being a member of the Center for Drug Evaluation for the US Food and Drug Administration Advisory Committee.

Professor Anita Zaidi reported a significant research interest in the management of typhoid fever, and had been the senior author of Cochrane systematic reviews on this topic. She also reported support from the Novartis Vaccine Foundation to her department, for studies on the immunogenicity of conjugate typhoid vaccine.

Professor David Ofori-Adjei reported being the team leader for monitoring and evaluation of a Pfizer-sponsored mobilize against malaria project in Ghana. He was asked not to contribute to recommendations on antimalarials.

Professor Hany Abdel-Aleem, Dr Lisa A Bero, Professor Abdol Majid Cheraghali, Professor Rohini Fernandopulle, and Dr Lenita Wannmacher reported no conflicts of interest.

Temporary Advisers reported the following interests:

Dr Agnès Saint-Raymond reported being a full-time employee of the European Medicines Agency.

Professor Jennifer Welbeck reported no conflict of interest.

1. Introduction

The 18th meeting of the WHO Expert Committee on the Selection and Use of Essential Medicines was held from 21 to 25 March 2011, in Accra, Ghana.

The meeting was opened by the WHO Representative in Ghana on behalf of the Director-General of the World Health Organization (WHO). The WHO Representative noted that this is the first time a WHO Expert Committee has met outside of Geneva and thanked the Ghana Ministry of Health for agreeing to allow the meeting to be held in Accra.

The WHO Representative noted that Expert Committee members are selected from panels of experts that are nominated from many organizations and governments. Expert Panel and Committee members are required to provide advice as individuals, however, and may not take directions from any external organization or government.

Dr Clive Ondari welcomed members on behalf of the Department of Essential Medicines and Pharmaceutical Policies and noted that this was an unique event, being the first Expert Committee meeting to be held outside of WHO Headquarters in Geneva.

2. Open session

The open session was attended by a variety of interested parties, as well as representatives and observers from the Ghana Ministry of Health. The Secretariat provided a brief update on activities since the last meeting of the Expert Committee and highlighted issues to be addressed during the 18th Expert Committee meeting.

The following comments on agenda items were noted.

1. Comments were submitted in writing by Médecins Sans Frontières on malaria treatment, miltefosine, succimer, antiretroviral medicines, neglected diseases in children, and on the treatment of tuberculosis (TB) in children. An additional comment on the last subject was also submitted.
2. A statement of support on the inclusion of misoprostol for the prevention of postpartum haemorrhage, presented by Professor SWK Adadevoh (Ghana).

The following additional comments from participants were provided to the Committee.

1. A statement of support for the inclusion of misoprostol for the prevention of postpartum haemorrhage, by Professor A Gessessew (Ethiopia).

3. Review of Report of supplementary session, January 2010: Other antiviral medicines

A Supplementary Meeting of the WHO Expert Committee on the Selection and Use of Essential Medicines took place in Geneva on 15 January 2010, to consider whether oseltamivir and zanamivir should be added to the EML in the context of the influenza A (H1N1) pandemic. Applications for inclusion of these medicines had previously been considered in 2009, and both had been rejected.

At the January 2010 meeting,[1] the Committee noted that:

> The evidence from randomized clinical trials for all antivirals has not changed substantially since March 2009. However, there has been more experience of the use of oseltamivir since the declaration of the pandemic, and the observational data resulting from this use provide some estimates of effectiveness. Since March 2009, there is also more evidence of the relative safety of oseltamivir in a range of patient and age groups, with no evidence of harm. The updated WHO recommendations concerning use of oseltamivir for treatment of seriously ill patients or those in higher-risk groups are based on these data. Oseltamivir resistance has been described, very rarely, for the current pandemic H1N1 strain. In these cases, the virus has remained susceptible to zanamivir. However, there remain concerns that increasing use of antivirals will lead to increased resistance.
>
> Based on the available evidence of the potential benefit of oseltamivir in specific patient groups and the expected prevalence of pandemic H1N1 in the coming seasons, the Expert Committee agreed to add this medicine to the Core List. The Committee specified that the List should include the following notes: oseltamivir should be used only in compliance with the WHO treatment guidelines, i.e. (1) for treatment of patients with severe or progressive clinical illness with confirmed or suspected influenza pandemic (H1N1) 2009, (2) for the treatment of patients with confirmed or suspected but uncomplicated illness due to pandemic influenza virus infection who were in higher risk groups, most notably for pregnant women and children under 2 years of age.
>
> Oseltamivir will be listed in the following dosage forms:
>
> - Capsule: 30 mg; 45 mg; 75 mg.
> - Oral powder: 12 mg/ml.

1 http://www.who.int/selection_medicines/committees/expert/emergency_session/unedited_Emergency_report.pdf.

Zanamavir, amantadine, and rimantadine were also considered by the Committee but were not added to the List.

The Committee noted the report of the Supplementary Session. The Committee then reviewed the listing of oseltamivir, given that the pandemic was declared over on 10 August 2010. Since that time, WHO has started the process of updating the clinical guidelines to consolidate information on management of influenza, and has commissioned an independent full review of the clinical evidence. The preliminary report of this review was provided in confidence to the Committee prior to submission for publication. Expert reviews for this meeting were provided by Dr Lisa A Bero and Mr Andy Gray.

The Committee noted that there were no new published randomized trials of any of the four available antivirals and also noted the publication of a protocol for a Cochrane Review of unpublished data from randomized controlled trials (RCTs), see Annex 5. The review provided to the Committee of the observational studies suggests that oseltamivir treatment is associated with a statistically significant reduction in mortality (OR 0.28; 95% CI 0.17–0.47) with similar trends seen for other outcomes (hospitalization, complications). The meta-analysis of critical adverse events such as neuropsychiatric events, skin reactions, and movement disorders shows increased events in patients treated with oseltamivir. The evidence, however, was described as low or very low quality, and the possibility for publication bias was noted. Data for zanamivir, amantadine, and rimantadine were also summarized, as were the very limited data for comparative effectiveness.

The Committee noted the comments from the WHO Global Influenza Programme concerning the use of oseltamivir and decided to confirm the decision of the Supplementary Session of the Expert Committee. The Committee also noted the lack of appropriate data to guide the management of illness in children aged less than 1 year, noting that children aged less than 2 years were considered a particular risk group, and recommended that this issue be prioritized by WHO.

The Committee ratified the report of the between-sessions meeting and decided to retain oseltamivir on the WHO Model Lists of Essential Medicines (EMLs); see Annexes 1–4. The Committee decided that further specific review of this decision was not needed. The Committee also noted the usefulness of the between-sessions meeting and recommended that it be used in the future as needed.

4. General items

1: IUPHAR – report on clinical pharmacology

In 1970, WHO published a report of a WHO Study Group on clinical pharmacology, detailing its scope, organization, and training requirements. The stated purpose of that report was to define the discipline of clinical pharmacology and to outline how it could help to improve the use of drugs in the delivery of health care. As a report of a formal Study Group, it was published as a WHO Technical Report.

The Committee noted that there has been discussion over the past five years about the potential for updating this document. The reasons for updating it would be to provide further guidance on the role of clinical pharmacology in pharmaceutical policy development and rational use of medicines, as well as potentially promoting the role of the discipline in health care systems. The International Union of Basic and Clinical Pharmacology (IUPHAR) Working Group prepared an updated paper entitled *Clinical pharmacology in research, teaching and health care* published in the journal *Basic and Clinical Pharmacology & Toxicology* (*1*).

The Committee noted the comments received on the report. It also noted the recent WHO guidelines most relevant to definitions of particular specialties: the WHO Guidelines on Task Shifting. There are no other current WHO documents that describe a profession or specialty role. The Committee also noted the comments from several experts concerning the challenges in implementing clinical pharmacology activities and the roles assigned to clinical pharmacology as a discipline.

The Committee therefore decided to note the existing publication by IUPHAR as an important reference on the role of clinical pharmacology in clinical care and public health and also to note its potential value in supporting pharmaceutical sector development. The Committee also noted the additional papers submitted in respect of paediatric clinical pharmacology and geriatric clinical pharmacology. The Committee endorsed the need for persons with appropriate competencies in this area to have access to health systems, particularly to drive the implementation of the Essential Medicines concept in resource-constrained settings.

2: How to develop a national essential medicines list

The Committee noted the draft document *How to develop a national essential medicines list* prepared by the WHO Secretariat and also the comments provided by Professor Abdol Majid Cheraghali. The Committee noted the importance of having such guidance and therefore recommended that further revisions were needed. The need for further consultation with potential users of the guidance was emphasized.

3: Rational use of medicines – future strategies and directions

The Committee noted the report from the Secretariat summarizing the progress and reports on rational use of medicines since the WHO Resolution WHA60.16 in 2007. The Committee suggested the following for consideration in the development of future WHO activities in this area:

- close coordination between processes for the development of standard treatment guidelines and efforts to improve quality use of medicines;
- continued emphasis on the inclusion of the essential medicines concept in undergraduate and post-graduate medical, pharmacy, and nursing curricula;
- greater emphasis on the effective utilization of drug and therapeutics committees at regional, district, and facility levels;
- greater emphasis on measurement and monitoring of medicines use, in order to target interventions to context-specific needs; and
- greater emphasis on the effect of social or national health insurance systems on the quality of medicines used.

The Committee suggested that further development and expansion of projects targeting elements of antimicrobial stewardship would provide a useful globally-applicable target area for WHO's efforts, which can include countries at all levels of development. It was emphasized that efforts to address the quality of medicines used need to be directed at more than just prescribers, but target all aspects of medicines use.

4: Updated list of missing drug formulations for HIV treatment

At its 2009 meeting the Committee considered a list of 'missing essential medicines' for HIV, proposed by UNITAID and WHO, and recommended that this list be regularly reviewed and updated. The purpose of this list was in part to assist the development of a priority list of molecules for the Medicines Patent Pool, which has now been established and funded by UNITAID as a separate entity.

The WHO HIV/AIDS Department convened a prioritization exercise in April 2011 to produce a list of missing essential medicines for HIV; this new list will inform future efforts within the Medicines Patent Pool and in pharmaceutical development.

The Committee expressed support for the maintenance of a missing essential medicines list, including but not limited to medicines for children, and those covering priority needs worldwide.

5: Guidance on the extemporaneous preparation of medicines for children (draft for consultation)

The Committee noted the preliminary draft of guidance on extemporaneous preparation of medicines for children, commissioned by WHO.

The Committee accepted that there may be situations where extemporaneous preparation of medicines for children is necessary, but was concerned about the risks of inappropriate preparations. The Committee also considered the risks of diverting efforts aimed at the development of age-appropriate dosage forms for children and indicated that WHO endorsement of extemporaneous use should not be seen, in any way, as indicating a lack of need for commercially available paediatric dosage forms. The Committee raised concerns about potential conflicting signals arising from a WHO publication that might appear to endorse wider use of manipulation of adult dosage forms for children.

Notwithstanding these concerns, the Committee agreed that the document should be finalized for publication as a time-limited guidance that addresses the current need for advice, including review by the Expert Committee on the Specification of Pharmaceuticals. Consideration may be given to publication of this guidance document by an organization other than WHO.

6: Review of proposed medical module for inpatient management of severe acute malnutrition with medical complications in children

The Committee reviewed the submission from the Health Action in Crises (HAC) cluster, concerning a proposed list of medicines to be provided as an emergency kit for inpatient management of children with acute medical complications and severe malnutrition.

The Committee questioned the need for such a kit, given the existence of the *Interagency emergency health kit* and suggested that discussions within the Interagency Pharmaceutical Coordination Group were needed. The Committee was advised of the experience of Aga Khan Hospital in managing the transition from emergency responses to ongoing hospital supply following the floods in Sind province, Pakistan. It would be challenging to devise a globally-relevant list to address the very specific needs that may arise in different populations and settings.

The Committee considered the medicines on the proposed list, and raised the issue of lack of data in respect of the differences in pharmacokinetics and responses to medicines in children with different types of acute or chronic malnutrition. The Committee noted that there were several medicines proposed for the list that did not appear on the current WHO Model List of Essential Medicines for Children (EMLc). The Committee suggested that a subgroup be identified to consider whether a list of this nature was needed. If the decision was that such a list was both needed and possible, a working group drawn from the Expert Panel on Drug Evaluation should be tasked with its development.

7: Review of application process

At the end of the meeting, the Committee reviewed its experience of evaluating the applications that had been submitted. The Committee was concerned that some applications did not provide all relevant published and unpublished data, and noted that at a minimum, applications should provide a comprehensive search strategy to identify relevant clinical data and should present all published data, or justify fully any exclusion. Some applications considered at the meeting that had been submitted by commercial organizations were clearly too selective and were based on dossiers submitted to regulatory authorities, without appropriate consideration of publicly accessible data from peer-reviewed publications. Further, the Committee was concerned that applications submitted by manufacturers might not include all data available from unpublished studies, and identified several examples where the data that were provided were not presented in formats that allowed correct and complete interpretation (e.g. presentation of point estimates as percentage only without numbers of confidence intervals). It was also difficult to correctly identify publications based on unpublished trials and sometimes only pooled data without the individual study results were provided.

The Committee recommended that it should have access to all data provided to WHO relating to medicines on its agenda, including 'confidential data' provided to other WHO committees. Otherwise it could not fully assess an application and would have no choice but to defer it. The Secretariat was asked to consider more critical screening of applications that failed to include data from a comprehensive search of available clinical evidence of efficacy and safety. The Committee requested the Secretariat to review the trends in applications from manufacturers and other sources over time, so that proposals for revision of the standard procedures and applications forms can be considered.

8: Essential medicines that can be used in neonates

The Committee noted that as a result of the updates to the EMLc, Appendix B of the *WHO Technical Report Series*, No. 958 needed to be amended to reflect the additions and deletions. The updated list is the Appendix to Annex 2.

5. Applications only for paediatric medicines

Section 2: Analgesics, antipyretic medicines, non-steroidal anti-inflammatory medicines (NSAIMs), medicines used to treat gout, and disease-modifying agents in rheumatoid disorders (DMARDs)

Section 2.1: Non-opioids and non-steroidal anti-inflammatory medicines (NSAIMs)

Ibuprofen (review) – Children

At its 2009 meeting, the Committee requested a review of ibuprofen use in children for the treatment of fever and pain. The current EMLc includes ibuprofen, as tablet, for the treatment of pain and fever in infants aged more than 3 months, and for the treatment of acute attacks of migraine, and ibuprofen as oral liquid or tablet for palliative care (treatment of bone pain). A review was prepared for the Committee by Mr Andy Gray, University of KwaZulu-Natal, South Africa. Expert reviews were provided by Dr Lisa A Bero and Professor Anita Zaidi.

The Committee noted that the review included evidence from three systematic reviews and RCTs in the treatment of pain and fever. The Committee considered the first systematic review (*2*) which analysed efficacy and safety data for both ibuprofen and paracetamol in children and adults. Based on English language publications only, there were 18 prospective or retrospective studies in infants, children, and adolescents. Eleven studies found no difference in analgesic efficacy between paracetamol and ibuprofen and seven reported superiority for ibuprofen. The estimate of standardized mean difference in pain measurement was 0.28 (95% CI 0.1–0.46) in favour of ibuprofen (within 2 hours of dosing).

The effect on fever was analysed in 30 studies; 15 concluded that ibuprofen was superior to paracetamol and 15 showed no difference. The Committee noted that of the 7 RCTs involving 576 participants, only 1 included children aged 2 to 14 years. The estimate of standardized mean difference in fever from these seven trials was 0.26 (95% CI 0.1–0.41) in favour of ibuprofen (within 4 hrs of dosing).

Two additional studies were considered to identify the benefit of either paracetamol or ibuprofen as antipyretics. One was a meta-analysis of animal studies of antipyretics used in influenza (*3*), which suggested an increase in mortality in influenza-infected animals associated with antipyretic use (OR 1.34; 95% CI 1.04–1.73). The second study, a RCT of antipyretics in 231 children aged 4 months to 4 years (mean 1.7 years) showed no efficacy of antipyretics on the prevention of febrile seizures, and no efficacy on fever accompanying febrile seizures. The trial used maximum recommended doses of antipyretics (rectal diclofenac or placebo as first line, then oral ibuprofen, paracetamol, or placebo) and confirmed previous data on the lack of efficacy on febrile seizures prevention (*4*).

The Committee also considered the evidence of safety from 31 studies from the systematic review (*2*). A single trial concluded that paracetamol was better tolerated and all others showed no difference between paracetamol and ibuprofen. A review (*5*) of 24 RCTs and 12 observational studies showed no significant difference between ibuprofen and paracetamol for adverse events requiring discontinuation, and systemic reactions (RR 0.54; 95% CI 0.17–1.71 and RR 1.03; 95% CI 0.98–1.10, respectively).

The Committee considered that the short use of ibuprofen in these indications may explain the lack of toxicity, as NSAIMs toxicity is increased by longer-term use, higher doses, and increased age and paracetamol liver toxicity is due to overdosing (intentional or not).

Asthma-related symptoms were specifically analysed by Kanabar et al. (*6*), who concluded that there might be a protective effect of ibuprofen compared to paracetamol.

The Committee noted that the median cost of a 100-ml bottle of paracetamol is US$ 0.39 while that of ibuprofen would be US$ 0.87. The Committee also noted that the new WHO treatment guidelines on the management of persistent pain in children include recommendations for use of ibuprofen.

The Committee noted that administration of antipyretics is established practice, but that there is no compelling evidence of clinical benefit from the treatment of fever. There is concern that reduction of fever may itself be associated with possible harm. The Committee also noted that there may be adverse effects associated with either paracetamol or ibuprofen, and therefore decisions to treat fever in children would need to take account of the trade-off between benefits and harms.

The Committee recommended including ibuprofen suspension (200 mg/5 ml) for the treatment of pain as a safe alternative to paracetamol, noting that there are no data to support its use in infants aged less than 3 months. The Committee noted the need for flexible oral solid dosage forms, suitable for children, but decided to list the oral liquid form at this time, due to availability and cost.

Section 2.2: Opioid analgesics

Codeine (deletion) – Children

An application was prepared by Dr Barbara Milani, Technical Officer, Department of Essential Medicines and Pharmaceutical Policies, WHO Secretariat, for the deletion of codeine from Section 2.2 of the Model List of Essential Medicines for Children.

An expert review was prepared by Professor Abdol Majid Cheraghali.

The Committee was informed that the WHO guidelines on the pharmacological treatment of persisting pain in children with medical illnesses have recently been updated. The new guidelines recommend the use of paracetamol or ibuprofen, followed by morphine if pain has not been adequately controlled. Codeine is no longer recommended. The Committee noted that in children aged less than 5 years, the enzyme required to convert codeine to its active metabolite, morphine, is estimated to be no higher than 25% of adult values and as a result the analgesic effect of codeine is low or absent in neonates and young children (*7*). The Committee also noted that there is considerable pharmacogenetic variability among populations; treatment with codeine is ineffective in poor metabolizers and potentially toxic in fast and extensive metabolizers. Codeine therefore should not be regarded as an adequate substitute for morphine. The Committee considered indirect evidence from one RCT (*8*) that suggests codeine is no better than ibuprofen or paracetamol in terms of efficacy and safety for the treatment of musculoskeletal trauma in children.

The Committee therefore recommended the deletion of codeine from Section 2.2 of the Model List of Essential Medicines for Children due to evidence indicating that the analgesic effect is low or absent in neonates and young children; evidence of considerable pharmacogenetic variability among populations, making its efficacy and safety questionable in an unpredictable proportion of the paediatric population; and low-quality evidence indicating that it is not safer or more efficacious than paracetamol or ibuprofen for the treatment of musculoskeletal trauma in children. The Committee also noted the need to improve access to appropriate analgesics, especially morphine, in all settings.

Further, the Committee recommended that the inclusion of codeine 30 mg in the EML for adults be reviewed.

Section 2.4: Disease-modifying agents used in rheumatoid disorders

Methotrexate, sulfasalazine, azathioprine, leflunomide, hydroxychloroquine, mycophenolate, and cyclosporine (review) – Children

At its 2009 meeting, the Committee had requested a review of the medicines needed for the treatment of juvenile idiopathic arthritis (JIA) in children, as it did not endorse any of the medicines currently listed. The current EMLc includes acetylsalicylic acid to treat systemic onset JIA, Kawasaki disease, and rheumatic fever (Complementary List), as well as immunoglobulins (intravenous Ig) for Kawasaki disease.

A review was prepared by P Gowdie (Royal Children's Hospital, Melbourne, Australia) to identify priority rheumatic conditions in children, treatment options, evidence for efficacy and safety, and to make recommendations for the inclusion of medicines. Professor Rohini Fernandopulle and Dr Lenita Wannmacher provided expert reviews.

The Committee noted that the most frequent condition in children is JIA, with three main forms: systemic onset, polyarticular, and oligo-monoarticular. Other conditions of interest are juvenile dermatomyositis/polymyositis (JDM), and systemic lupus erythematosus (SLE), but these are infrequent in children. Other chronic arthritic diseases affecting children such as acute rheumatic fever, Lyme disease, post-streptococcal reactive arthritis, Kawasaki disease, and other vasculitides were not discussed in the application.

The Committee noted that the following pharmacological classes were used: NSAIMs for the management of symptoms; corticosteroids at immunosuppressive doses (especially for paediatric SLE and JDM); and DMARDs which include methotrexate, cyclophosphamide, azathioprine, cyclosporine, mycophenolate, leflunomide, sulfasalazine, and chloroquine or hydroxychloroquine. DMARDs aim to control disease activity, prevent irreversible organ damage, and decrease the burden of the disease or steroid treatment.

The Committee first considered whether these conditions represent a priority health problem for the population. Estimates of prevalence are available for JIA in developed countries (from 7 to 401 per 100 000 children) and this condition can produce a high burden of disease if it continues into adulthood with severe disability or the need for joint replacement. Juvenile dermatomyositis, on the other hand, is a rare disease and if treated appropriately with high doses of steroids, immunosuppressants and supportive care, can result in little disability. The prevalence of paediatric SLE, a chronic, life-threatening disease, ranges between 0.36 and 0.9 per 100 000 children. The Committee noted the lack of specific data in children affected by chronic arthritis or inflammatory systemic diseases in developing countries.

The Committee evaluated the evidence provided in the review for each of the medicines. A summary of the considerations is provided in Table 1 and full details of the clinical evidence are in the application.

Methotrexate

The Committee noted that the use of methotrexate (MTX) in children requires monitoring, in particular of liver enzymes, on a regular basis. The Committee noted the risk of serious adverse effects associated with inadvertent daily dosing of MTX instead of weekly. Such mistakes can be due to prescribing errors (commonly seen at transfers between sites of care), dispensing errors, and patient errors.

The Committee concluded that methotrexate should be included in the Complementary List of the EMLc, based on the evidence of efficacy and safety available in children.

Table 1
Review of DMARDs

Medicine	Indications	Summary of evidence	Dosage
Methotrexate (MTX)	Juvenile idiopathic arthritis (JIA), juvenile dermatomyositis/ polymyositis (JDM), uveitis, systemic lupus erythematosus (SLE), localized scleroderma and vasculitis	JIA Cochrane Review: 2 randomized controlled trials (RCTs) (165 patients) MTX effective on patient-centred disability, 3–23% greater with MTX than with placebo (*12*), a meta-analysis (*13*) a large RCT (*14*). JDM Use based on expert consensus (*15*) and 3 retrospective studies showing shorter discontinuation of steroids and reduced cumulative dose. Short- and long-term data suggest that MTX is a safe drug in the paediatric population (*16*, *17*).	Tablet 2.5 mg (0.0365/tab-cap to 0.1327/tab-cap)
Leflunomide	JIA	Several RCTs: leflunomide and MTX both produced clinical improvement; more patients on MTX met the primary end-point (ACR Pediatric 30 response) than on leflunomide (89% vs 68%, respectively) (*18*). Common adverse effects: headache, rash, and alopecia; liver abnormalities can occur. Teratogenic and requires liver function monitoring.	—
Sulfasalazine (SAS)	JIA	Two small RCTs showed superiority over placebo, but no significant difference with chloroquine. More adverse effects in the SAS group (*19*, *20*).	Tablet 500 mg (0.0865/tab-cap to 0.2349/tab-cap)

continues

Table 1 *continued*

Medicine	Indications	Summary of evidence	Dosage
Sulfasalazine (SAS)	JIA	A third trial showed no efficacy of SAS over placebo (n=33) (*21*). SAS does not have consistent efficacy across subtypes of JIA (poor tolerance). Adverse effects include rash, gastrointestinal symptoms and leucopenia, resulting in discontinuation in up to 30% of patients (*19*). Liver abnormalities and serious, even fatal, liver toxicity is associated with the DRESS syndrome (Drug Reaction with Eosinophilia and Systemic Symptoms). Agranulocytosis has been reported in 1% of patients.	Tablet 500 mg (0.0865/tab-cap to 0.2349/tab-cap)
Cyclosporine (CyA)	JIA	Non-RCTs A prospective open trial over 10 years in 34 children with systemic onset JIA showed no effect on arthritis, and poor tolerance with 76% withdrawals (15/34 children for lack of efficacy and 9/34 for adverse effects) (*22*). Renal toxicity and hypertension are the most common adverse effects of CyA and main causes for withdrawal of therapy (*23*); other adverse effects include hypertrichosis, gingival hyperplasia, gastrointestinal (GI) disturbances, tremor, paresthesias, hepatic dysfunction and bone marrow suppression. Risk of secondary malignancies is increased at high doses. Nephrotoxicity is increased when combining CyA with other nephrotoxic medicines such as NSAIMS. CyA use requires monitoring of blood pressure, and renal function.	Tablet 25 mg (0.2860/tab-cap to 0.3576/tab-cap) Solution 100 mg/ml (1.1538/ml to 4.0789/ml)

continues

Table 1 *continued*

Medicine	Indications	Summary of evidence	Dosage
Azathioprine (AZA)	Refractory JIA, SLE	Refractory JIA – single RCT of AZA in 32 children with JIA failed to show efficacy over placebo (*24*). Observational studies suggest clinical and laboratory improvements (*25*) of paediatric SLE; and a small observational study suggested survival gains (*26*). Safety data: frequent GI symptoms in up to 12% of patients receiving AZA, less common pancreatitis, liver toxicity, interstitial pneumonitis, and serious dose-dependent adverse effects on bone marrow (genetically low thiopurine methyltransferase TMTP activity).	Tablet 50 mg (0.1379/tab to 0.1724 /tab)
Hydroxychloroquine (HCQ)	JIA	JIA 2 RCTs: (*27, 28*) HCQ (6 mg/kg) vs penicillamine in 162 patients: no significant difference; and in 72 patients, HCQ was not more efficacious than gold or penicillamine. Rheumatoid arthritis (RA): a Cochrane Review comparing HCQ to placebo in adult patients with rheumatoid arthritis revealed an overall moderate effect and low toxicity profile (*29*).	Tablet 200 mg (0.1100 /tab-cap to 0.1986 /tab-cap)

Hydroxychloroquine

For hydroxychloroquine (HCQ), currently not in the EML, the Committee considered that there is evidence for efficacy and safety in adult SLE: a RCT (Canadian Hydroxychloroquine Study Group) showed that adult patients assigned to the placebo group had a significantly higher relative risk of flare and shorter time to flare compared to those patients who continued HCQ; and a recent systematic review of 95 articles (all ages) that concluded that there was evidence that antimalarials used in lupus prevent lupus flares and increase long-term survival of patients with SLE, and moderate evidence of protection against irreversible organ damage, thrombosis, and bone mass loss, with infrequent and reversible toxicity (*9*). The low cost of HCQ is an advantage for a systematic prescription in SLE patients.

The Committee also noted that the Childhood Arthritis and Rheumatology Research Alliance (CARRA) recommends hydroxychloroquine for milder cases of juvenile dermatomyositis and cases mainly characterized by rash (*10*). In children the recommended dose is 3–5 mg/kg per day with a maximum of 400 mg (as once or twice daily with food).

The Committee noted that HCQ is generally safe, including during pregnancy and breastfeeding. Common adverse effects include gastrointestinal (GI) and central nervous system (CNS) disturbances. The most serious irreversible adverse effect, however, is retinal (macular) toxicity, which can lead to blindness. The maximum safe daily dose in adults is 6.5 mg/kg, but is not defined in children (European Union, EU, product information). Detection of early retinal changes requires yearly monitoring and, if discovered, should lead to discontinuation of HCQ.

The Committee considered that there is evidence of effectiveness for hydroxychloroquine in SLE and recommended its inclusion in the EMLc Complementary List with availability of ophthalmologic monitoring as a condition for its use. A review in respect of adults would be prepared for the next meeting.

Leflunomide, sulfasalazine, azothiaprine, cyclosporine, mycophenolate

The Committee considered that although the review recommended the inclusion of leflunomide, it appears less effective than methotrexate with a similar safety profile and therefore did not recommend its inclusion in the Model List. Similarly, despite the recommendation made in the review, the Committee considered that the evidence supporting the use of sulfasalazine and azothiaprine in JIA was too limited and indicated poor tolerance and the need for regular monitoring to detect potentially serious adverse effects. The

Committee also considered that the evidence of efficacy for cyclosporin was insufficient to recommend inclusion.

Mycophenolate was not addressed in the application but commented upon by the second reviewer. The Committee noted that there is limited evidence in children indicating the possibility to reduce steroid doses (*11*) but no evidence of benefits over cyclophosphamide in adults with lupus nephritis. The Committee considered that there was insufficient evidence of effectiveness and safety to support inclusion in the EMLc.

Lastly, the Committee signalled the need for a review of the order of chloroquine versus hydroxychloroquine as a DMARD in adults.

Section 4: Antidotes and other substances used in poisonings

Section 4.2: Specific

Oral iron chelation therapy (review) – Children

In 2009, the Expert Committee requested a review of iron chelators for children. The current EMLc includes deferoxamine only, for parenteral use. Dr A Algren prepared the review for the Committee.

Expert reviews were provided by Dr Gregory L Kearns and Dr Lisa A Bero.

The Committee noted a recent review of iron chelators (*30*).

Acute iron intoxication can occur in both adults and children and can be fatal. Treatment includes supportive care, and parenteral deferoxamine. Chronic iron overload is due mainly to repeat transfusions, in patients with haemoglobinopathies. Other conditions requiring repeat transfusions include myelodysplastic syndromes, and (more rarely) haemochromatosis. Long-term consequences of chronic iron overload include multiple organ dysfunction (heart, liver, and endocrine), and/or failure, and death. Heart failure due to iron myocardiopathy is the main cause of death in thalassaemia patients.

The Committee reviewed the evidence available for acute iron poisoning. Two studies in volunteers showed that iron removal was possible with high doses of oral deferoxamine. The Committee noted that a recent placebo-controlled trial of deferasirox (20 mg/kg) showed iron elimination after a 5 mg/kg iron dose in volunteers (*31*).

A systematic review of observational and prospective studies suggests beneficial effects of deferoxamine on morbidity (notably cardiac disease and liver iron overload) and mortality, including with subcutaneous use (*32–37*). In sickle-cell disease, evidence is more limited but supports the use of deferoxamine. Deferoxamine has adverse effects on growth and maturation, auditory, and ophthalmic function. The Committee considered that the main limitation of deferoxamine was however the need for prolonged parenteral administration, and a trial showed less compliance with parenteral deferoxamine than oral deferiprone (*38*).

The Committee noted that the evidence supporting use of deferiprone comprises small trials – mostly observational including both adults and children summarized in a Cochrane Review from 2007 (10 trials including 398 participants). The dose used in trials was generally 75 mg/kg per day, and reported adverse effects included neutropaenia and agranulocytosis, which require weekly monitoring of blood cell counts. Gastrointestinal symptoms are common and knee arthralgias are reversible. Neurological signs at doses above 100 mg/kg have been reported in children. The use of the combination of deferiprone and deferoxamine was found to be more effective than single agents with promising results of normalization of ferritinaemia (*39*). The review concluded that there was no consistent effect on reduction of iron overload among various treatments. Deferoxamine was more effective on iron excretion in three of four trials. Trials did not report on mortality or end organ damage (*38*). The Committee concluded that the evidence supporting the effectiveness of deferiprone was insufficient.

The evidence of effectiveness of deferasirox is more recent and of better quality than is the case for deferiprone. The Committee noted a large non-randomized uncontrolled prospective company-sponsored trial in 192 patients (64 aged less than 16 years), which showed a statistically significant decrease in cardiac iron (assessed by MRI) after one year of treatment (*40*). A Cochrane Review of deferasirox in sickle-cell disease identified only one study and concluded that deferasirox appeared to be as effective as deferoxamine, but important outcomes were missing. No data are available to support the current use of deferasirox in myelodysplastic syndromes.

The Committee noted that deferasirox has renal adverse effects, which require regular monitoring of renal function. Dose-dependent increases in serum creatinine, which may occur in up to 36% of patients, may not always be reversible. Tubulopathy has also been reported in children with thalassaemia (EU product information).

The Committee considered the costs of deferoxamine, including laboratory monitoring cost, adverse effects and/or worsening of underlying disease as a result of non-compliance, hospitalization, parenteral injections, need for carer, and missed school days. The cost of deferasirox treatment may be 2–3 times more than that of deferoxamine, and the cost of deferiprone could be twice that of deferoxamine. The Committee noted that several reports suggest that deferasirox therapy is more cost effective than traditional deferoxamine therapy but considered that a truly unbiased cost comparison between deferiprone and deferasirox has not been published. The Committee noted that reports of costs analysis highlight variation in acquisition costs and resources used (*41*). The acquisition cost of deferasirox is an important barrier to access, but adherence to infused deferoxamine is also problematic and administration costs also need to be considered.

Although noting the advantages of the oral route, the Committee did not recommend the inclusion of deferasirox in the EML and EMLc at this stage, but recommended adding an asterisk to deferoxamine, noting the alternative oral form (deferasirox 500 mg dispersible oral solid dosage form) is available. As an antidote, deferoxamine should be listed on the Complementary List due to the level of care required for its safe use.

Oral lead chelation therapy (review) – Children
Sodium calcium edetate and penicillamine (review) – Children

The Committee requested a review of medicines used for lead chelation in children, with particular focus on sodium calcium edetate and penicillamine, but with potential inclusion of oral succimer. The application was prepared by Dr J Lowry.

Expert reviews were provided by Dr Gregory L Kearns and Dr Lisa A Bero for the review on lead chelation, and Dr Kalle Hoppu and Professor Anita Zaidi for sodium calcium edentate and penicillamine.

The current EMLc includes dimercaprol, sodium calcium edetate, both used parenterally, and oral penicillamine.

The Committee acknowledged that lead poisoning is a common and serious poisoning. Most children with lead poisoning are in developing countries, where increased risks (e.g. iron deficiency) and increased exposure to lead are common. While primary prevention of lead poisoning is the most effective, chelation is used to decrease blood levels acutely on the basis of lead levels in blood. In symptomatic patients (encephalopathy), hospitalization is necessary and parenteral chelation is used.

The Committee reviewed the evidence available with parenteral and oral chelating medicines.

2,3-dimercapto-1-propanesulfonic acid (DMPS)

Racemic 2,3-dimercapto-1-propanesulfonic acid (DMPS) is a compound related to succimer and dimercaprol. It can be given orally or parenterally. The Committee noted that DMPS was used mostly in Germany and Russia for arsenic or mercury poisoning, and is not mentioned in guidelines on lead poisoning from the United States of America, United Kingdom of Great Britain and Northern Ireland, or France. The Committee considered that very few descriptive data exist on the dose in children; in one study the dose used safely in children was 200–400 mg/m^2 body surface area (*42*). Comparative animal data concluded that DMPS was less effective than sodium calcium edetate or succimer alone or in combination. DMPS is tolerated more poorly than succimer. The Committee concluded that the evidence of effectiveness and safe use of DMPS was insufficient.

Penicillamine

The Committee noted that there are very limited data on penicillamine, a chelator used primarily in Wilson disease. The most commonly used daily dose in the United States is 30 to 40 mg/kg or 600 to 750 mg/m^2 body surface area for one to six months. A retrospective study showed that penicillamine is more effective than placebo, decreasing blood lead by about 33%. In a comparative trial, it was as effective as dimercaprol or oral sodium calcium edetate given orally (*43*) but less effective than parenteral sodium calcium edetate. Penicillamine has major adverse effects (zinc depletion and its consequences, transient leukopenia, thrombocytopaenia, rash, enuresis, and abdominal pain) leading to discontinuation. The Committee noted that adverse effects affected 33% of 84 adult patients treated in a study. Children treated with 15 mg/kg per day may experience fewer adverse effects (*44*). While penicillamine has been used widely for lead chelation, its safety profile is a concern.

Sodium calcium edetate and dimercaprol

The Committee reviewed the evidence available for sodium calcium edetate and dimercaprol and noted that there is considerable experience but limited and low-quality evidence. Two prospective studies showed modest effect on lead excretion, but no benefit on IQ with sodium calcium edetate alone or combined with dimercaprol. The combination increased adverse effects. In contrast, a retrospective comparison of 18 children receiving either dimercaprol or sodium calcium edetate showed no residual intelligence deficit after about three years follow-up, and only a visual deficit more frequent in the dimercaprol group.

Dimercaprol is only recommended for use on the first day of treatment of acute poisoning in combination with calcium edetate disodium. The dose is 450 mg/m^2 per day and requires 4 to 6 intramuscular (IM) injections due to its short half-life.

One case series comparing sodium calcium edetate (IV, IM) and penicillamine in children, concluded that sodium calcium edetate was more effective on lead excretion than oral penicillamine and should be preferred in severe intoxications (>80 micrograms/dl) (*45*). The Committee considered safety data available for calcium edetate disodium. In a retrospective series, the most common adverse effect was renal toxicity. The Committee also noted reports of 3 deaths (2 in children) from hypocalcaemia-induced cardiac arrest, in the United States between 2003 and 2005, probably due to confusion with disodium edetate, normally indicated for the emergency treatment of hypercalcaemia.

The Committee concluded that, despite the low level of evidence to support its use, sodium calcium edetate had shown effectiveness for lead chelation in children.

The Committee considered cost–effectiveness data on different strategies of diagnostic and treatment by either sodium calcium edetate or penicillamine. Sodium calcium edetate dominated penicillamine in the incremental cost–effectiveness ratios (cost per quality-adjusted life year, QALY, and cost per case prevented), unless direct costs for inpatient treatment with sodium calcium edetate were included. The authors also concluded that, based on 200 000 children in the United States with blood lead levels >25 micrograms/dl, chelation therapy could prevent more than 45 000 cases of reading disability per year, resulting in savings of US$ 900 million in overall costs (*46*). No price data were available to the Committee from the International Price Indicator Guide[1] as the medicines reviewed are not listed there.

The Committee recommended that:

- sodium calcium edetate and dimercaprol be retained on the Complementary List of the EML and EMLc;
- dimercaprol is necessary for the initial phase of treatment (first day) to avoid increased toxicity from sodium calcium edetate but that its use should be restricted due to the need for multiple potentially painful and harmful IM injections per day;
- penicillamine be deleted from the EMLc, because of the higher risk of adverse effects in children; and
- DMPS not be included, due to insufficient evidence.

The Committee further recommended that the retention of penicillamine on the EML for adults be reviewed. Until this review is completed and considered, penicillamine will remain on the List.

[1] http://erc.msh.org/mainpage.cfm?file=1.0.htm&module=Dmp&language=English.

The Committee further recommended that Section 4.2 be restructured to clearly indicate the suggested division between items on the Core and Complementary Lists. Complementary designation was required because of the technical requirements of diagnosis and the potential for misuse of chelation therapy.

Succimer (new application) – Children

An application was prepared by Dr Volans, Dr Karalliedde and Ms Heather Wiseman, Medical Toxicology Information Services, Guy's and St Thomas' NHS Foundation Trust, United Kingdom, for the inclusion of succimer in the Model List. Listing is requested as an individual medicine.

Expert reviews were prepared by Professor Noël Cranswick and Professor David Ofori-Adjei. Comments were received from the Department for Evidence and Policy on Emerging Environmental Health issues, WHO; the European Association of Poisons Centres and Clinical Toxicologists, the American Academy of Clinical Toxicology, and Médecins Sans Frontières.

The Committee noted that succimer is recommended for children with moderate lead poisoning (45–69 micrograms/L), who can be protected from further exposure and have no signs of encephalopathy by international guidelines (*47–49*).

The Committee considered evidence from 4 RCTs (*50–53*), 3 observational studies (*54–56*), and 3 environmental studies (*57–59*) to support the safety and efficacy of succimer in children. The Committee noted that evidence for long-term effectiveness in children is limited and that no published studies have demonstrated an improvement in cognition, behaviour, or neuropsychological function in children given succimer compared to placebo. The Committee noted that compared with other antidotes for lead poisoning, succimer has a better adverse effect profile and causes less urinary loss of minerals.

The Committee noted that although there are no cost–effectiveness data for succimer compared to other lead chelators, the overall cost of treatment with succimer is likely to be lower because it can be administered orally and does not require hospitalization unlike parenteral chelators.

The Committee recommended the addition of succimer to the Model List for both children and adults, based on evidence of short-term efficacy, its favourable safety profile compared to other antidotes for lead poisoning, and the potential for cost savings because it can be administered orally and does not require hospitalization unlike parental antidotes. However, given the need for expert diagnosis and management of lead poisoning, it was decided to add this agent to the Complementary List.

Section 6: Anti-infective medicines

Neglected tropical diseases (review) – Children

In 2009, the Committee requested a review of the evidence supporting treatment of neglected tropical diseases in children. Neglected tropical diseases are a group of communicable diseases that affect around 1 billion people worldwide in 149 countries where these diseases are endemic. In at least 100 of these countries 2 or more diseases are endemic; in 30 others 6 or more are endemic. There are few new treatments available for the patients affected. The Secretariat commissioned the review which was prepared by Dr Rima Al-Saffer, Specialist Registrar, Paediatrics, United Kingdom and Dr Anna Louise Ridge, Technical Officer, Medicine Access and Rational Use, Department of Essential Medicines and Pharmaceutical Policies, WHO.

Expert reviews were provided Dr Lenita Wannmacher and Professor Anita Zaidi. Comments were received from the Department of Control of Neglected Tropical Diseases (NTDs), and from Médecins Sans Frontières.

The review focused on antischistosomal, antitrematode, anti-amoebic, antigiardiasis and antitrypanosomal medicines as these are the categories of medicines on the EMLc. It did not include consideration of dengue, rabies, trachoma, endemic treponematoses, leprosy, and echinococcosis.

The Committee noted that the review, while comprehensive, was limited to English-language articles, excluding potentially-relevant articles in Arabic, French, Portuguese, or Spanish, which may also reflect differences in strain susceptibility in different geographical regions. The review focuses on the following medicines: diethylcarbamazine (DEC), diloxanide, eflornithine, ivermectin, levamisole, mebendazole, melarsoprol, metronidazole, niclosamide, nifurtimox, oxamniquine, pentamidine, praziquantel, pyrantel, suramin sodium, and triclabendazole.

Section 6.1: Anthelminthics

For anthelminthics, the proposal from the expert reviews was to delete levamisole from the Model List as the evidence is limited and its efficacy in treating helminthic infections is less than that of albendazole, mebendazole, or pyrantel.

The NTD Department expressed the need to retain levamisole, while noting that its use alone is indeed becoming obsolete. It is listed in the 2006 guidelines, in combination with mebendazole, as a third-line option for the large-scale treatment of intestinal nematodiasis. The Committee noted the comments from the NTD Department but pointed out that the evidence does not support continuing the inclusion of levamisole and hence recommended that it be marked for consideration of deletion at the next meeting of the Committee. The Committee also added a note to the List that it is recommended that levamisole only be used in combination with other anthelminthics.

The Committee also decided to delete the square box symbol with mebendazole as all other relevant benzimidazoles are already included in the Model List as individual entries. It was noted that an oral liquid formulation of mebendazole is widely available, and that a more convenient age-appropriate dosage form than the chewable tablet was needed.

The expert reviews also recommended the deletion of niclosamide because of lack of evidence for efficacy and safety in children. The NTD Department expressed a wish to retain niclosamide for mass treatment programmes. However, noting the lack of evidence to support this view, the Committee recommended that niclosamide be marked for consideration of deletion at the next meeting of the Committee.

Section 6.2: Antifilarial medicines

For antifilarials, based on the evidence provided, the Committee decided to retain ivermectin and diethylcarbamazine, and add albendazole for combination therapy for both children and adults. There was no reason for diethylcarbamazine to be on the Complementary List especially since it is recommended by WHO guidelines as the drug of choice for mass drug administration in onchocerciasis-free areas. It was therefore moved to the Core List for both children and adults. The Committee recommended the deletion of suramin, for both children and adults, as it is no longer used for this indication.

Section 6.3: Antischistosomal and antitrematode medicines

For antischistosomal and antitrematode medicines, the Committee agreed to retain praziquantel and triclabendazole. The expert review proposed deletion of oxamniquine for children, due to its lower effectiveness and poor tolerability in comparison to adults, but the opinion of the NTD Department was that oxamniquine is the only currently available alternative (to praziquantel) treatment for schistosomiasis. Moreover, it is the only antischistosomal drug formally available as an appropriate paediatric formulation for use in children aged less than 4 years. Agreeing that this is an important consideration, the Committee decided to retain oxamniquine at this time. The Committee underlined the importance of identifying an effective and safe dose for oxamniquine in children, but also the need for an age-appropriate formulation of praziquantel.

Section 6.5: Antiprotozoal medicines

Section 6.5.1: Anti-amoebic and antigiardiasis medicines

For anti-amoebic and antigiardiasis medicines, no changes to the current Model List were recommended.

Section 6.5.2: Antileishmaniasis medicines

The Committee noted the report of the Expert Committee on the Control of Leishmaniases (*60*), dated 22–26 March 2010, but expressed concern that the recommendations of this Expert Committee were not explicitly linked with any sources of evidence. The existence of a global strategy for the control of neglected tropical diseases was also acknowledged (*61*). However, the Committee expressed concern about the lack of data in children, and the failure to adequately document the outcomes (including adverse effects) associated with mass administration of medicines in this group.

The application for inclusion of miltefosine is discussed in Section 6.5.2: Antileishmaniasis medicines of this report.

For African trypanosomiasis, the question was whether to delete suramin and melarsoprol. However, the Committee noted the previous review of this section (tabled in 2009) and decided to retain both products: suramin for treatment of first stage of *Trypanosoma brucei rhodesiense* African trypanosomiasis, and melarsoprol, for treatment of second stage disease in both African forms of the disease. Given the safety concerns, it was decided to move melarsoprol to the Complementary List for children. Melarsoprol needs to be retained for treatment of second stage disease, pending the outcome of ongoing trials comparing it to the combination of nifurtimox and eflornithine in children.

For American trypanosomiasis the proposal was to retain both benznidazole and nifurtimox for children. The Committee noted the response from the NTD Department, which proposed that nifurtimox should remain on the EMLc. The Committee therefore decided not to make any changes to this section of the List. The Committee, however, noted that a review of treatment options in Chagas disease is necessary, and suggested that this be done in coordination with the Pan American Health Organization.

In summary, the Committee noted with concern that there is a lack of progress in the development of paediatric treatment options for most neglected tropical diseases. Where recommendations for the management of children do exist, there is still a lack of data on pharmacokinetic and safety aspects. The Committee commented that there needed to be an evaluation of the impact of donation programmes that provide many of the current medicines used for the treatment of neglected tropical diseases on the development of new medicines or paediatric formulations.

Table 2 lists the data for the medicines referred to in the review of neglected tropical diseases in children, Sections 6.1 to 6.5.

Table 2
Studies conducted with anti-infective medicines

Drug name(s)	Studies reporting data for children	Efficacy data	Safety data	Doses reported	Formulation(s) reported
Mebendazole (MBZ)	10 studies [9 RCTs (*62–70*), 1 observational study (*71*); n=6856, age range 6 mos. to 70 yrs]. 2 studies included children <3 years (*62*, *65*).	All studies, except Flohr et al. (*63*) showed treatment with MBZ to be effective.	3 studies reported adverse events as an outcome (*62*, *64*, *65*). No serious adverse events reported. Main problems: nausea, abdominal distension, and discomfort.	200 mg tds; 500 mg od (most commonly used); 600 mg multiple doses.	Tablet 500 mg, chewable. No other information provided.
Levamisole (LVM)	3 studies [2 RCTs (*64*, *72*), 1 observational study (*73*); n=1633; age range 1 to 19 yrs]. 2 studies included children <4 yrs (*72*, *73*).	All studies showed efficacy based on reduction in egg counts. Albonico et al. (*68*) showed LVM to have smaller effect on egg clearance compared to MBZ or MBZ+LVM.	Adverse events occurring once in different patients (temperature rise, loose stools, convulsion) not reported to be directly related to LVM. No other adverse events reported.	<3 yrs: 40 mg 3–9 yrs: 60 mg >9 yrs: 80 mg	Tablet.

continues

Table 2 *continued*

Drug name(s)	Studies reporting data for children	Efficacy data	Safety data	Doses reported	Formulation(s) reported
Pyrantel (PYR)	4 studies [3 RCTS (*67, 68, 74*), 1 observational study (*74*)]: 3 (*68, 70, 74*) included only children (n=2074; age range 2 yrs to 10 yrs); 1 included adults and children (*67*) (n=147; age range 3 yrs to 70 yrs).	Effective in treating ascaris lumbricoides. Poor efficacy for treating hookworm infections. Higher cure rate than MBZ for trichuriasis infection, but less effective than albendazole.	None of the studies provided any information about adverse events/safety.	10 mg/kg/day 11 mg/kg/day 12.5 mg/kg/day 15–20 kg: 150 mg 21–30 kg: 300 mg 31–40 kg: 450 mg	Tablet.
Niclosamide	No	x	x	x	x
Diethyl-carbamizine (DEC)	6 studies [3 RCTs (*75–77*), 3 observational studies (*78–80*); n= >12000; age range 1 to 87 yrs].	All studies showed efficacy with a reduction in mf and antiginaemia.	Mild adverse events reported (nausea, vomiting, fever, headache). No cessation of treatment required.	6 mg/kg	No information reported.

continues

Table 2 *continued*

Drug name(s)	Studies reporting data for children	Efficacy data	Safety data	Doses reported	Formulation(s) reported
Ivermectin (IVM)	7 studies [4 RCTs (*77, 81–83*); 1 comparative field trial (*84*), 1 follow-up study (*85*), 1 safety study (*86*); n= 27632; age range 3 yrs to 87 yrs]. 2 studies included children <4 yrs (*85, 86*).	IVM treatment alone had lower mf clearance rates than combination therapy (IVM+albendazole).	No serious adverse events reported. Most frequently reported side-effects: headache, swellings, arthralgia, and fever.	Dose ranged from 150 mcg/kg to 400 mcg/kg.	3-mg tablet.
Praziquantel (PZQ)	13 studies [8 RCTs (*87–94*), 1 safety pilot study (*86*), 1 observational study (*95*), 2 clinical efficacy trial (*96, 97*), 1 quasi RCT (*98*)]. 8 studies included only children (*87, 89, 92–96*) (n = 5181; age range 4 yrs to 18 yrs). 5 studies included adults and children (*86, 88, 90, 91, 98*) (n= 5710; age range 7 yrs to 60 yrs).	Efficacy against *S. haematobium* (cure rate of 88.5%; egg reduction rate 98.2%). PZA more efficacious than niridazole, metrifonate, and placebo with ascorbic acid.	7 studies reported adverse events as an outcome (*88–91, 94, 96, 98*). Generally side-effects were mild and transient (dizziness, headache, abdominal pain, vomiting, diarrhoea). No cessation of treatment required.	20 mg/kg single oral dose. 20 mg/kg 2 oral doses. 20 mg/kg 3 oral doses. 40 mg/kg single dose. 60 mg/kg split dose 3 hrs apart.	200-mg tablet.

continues

Table 2 *continued*

Drug name(s)	Studies reporting data for children	Efficacy data	Safety data	Doses reported	Formulation(s) reported
Praziquantel (PZQ) **Additional information from unpublished studies**	5 observational studies 4 studies included preschool-age children (*99–102*) (n=1748; age range 1 month to 6 yrs). 1 study included primary-school children (*103*) (n=5700; age range 6 yrs to 12 yrs).	All studies showed efficacy of PZQ tablets and PZQ syrup with reduction in egg counts in consecutive stool/ urine samples. Efficacy of PZQ tablets shown to be greater than efficacy of PZQ syrup. PZQ treatment resulted in significant reduction in overall infection prevalence (29.5% to 5.68%) and infection intensity 19.7 to 1.39 eggs/10 ml urine.	All studies reported adverse events as an outcome. In general, PZA tablets and/ or syrup were well tolerated, with mild, transient side-effects (fatigue, dizziness, drowsiness, headache, loss of appetite, and stomach ache). 1 study showed symptoms were significantly higher among uninfected children compared to those with *S. mansoni*.	40 mg/kg 1–3 yrs: 518 mg; 1 tablet. >3–5 yrs: 740 mg; 1¼ tablet. >5–6yrs: 977 mg; 1⅔ tablet.	Tablet 600 mg (crushed and mixed with orange juice for younger children unable to swallow tablets; required dosage was broken into smaller pieces or crushed using mortar and pestle. A honey-based solution was added to make a suspension for some of the children). Syrup.

continues

Table 2 *continued*

Drug name(s)	Studies reporting data for children	Efficacy data	Safety data	Doses reported	Formulation(s) reported
Oxamniquine	9 studies [4 RCTs (*104–107*), 4 clinical efficacy trials (*108–111*), 1 follow-up study (*112*)]. 4 studies only included children (*104, 107, 108, 110*), (n=510; age range 2 yrs to 16 yrs). 5 studies included adults and children (*105, 106, 109, 111, 112*) (n>1261; age range 2 yrs to >20 yrs).	More effective at treating *S. mansoni* infection than *S. haematobium*. In children, lower doses not as successful in achieving cure as same doses in adults. Higher doses associated with an increase in adverse events. Better tolerated and more effective in adult groups.	Adverse events generally mild and transient. Dizziness, headache and drowsiness were the most commonly reported side-effects.	10 mg/kg bd for 1 day or 2 days 15 mg/kg single dose or bd for 1 day, 2 days or 8 days. 20 mg/kg single oral dose or bd for 1 day or 3 days. 800 mg/m^2/day in 2 divided doses (approx. 60 mg/kg). Optimal dose for children reported to be 30 mg/kg over 2 days (*104*) (n=162; age <15yrs).	Capsule. Suspension.
Triclabendazole	3 studies [1 pilot study (*113*), 1 case series (*114*), 1 community dose comparison study (*115*); n=184; age range 2 yrs to 62 yrs]. All studies included adults and children.	Cure rate with single dose 74.9%. Higher cure rate (93.9%) with 2 doses.	No significant adverse events. Good tolerability.	10 mg/kg od or bd.	Oral. No other information reported.

continues

Table 2 *continued*

Drug name(s)	Studies reporting data for children	Efficacy data	Safety data	Doses reported	Formulation(s) reported
Metronidazole	5 studies [1 RCT (*116*), 1 prospective open label randomized trial (*117*); 1 survey of efficacy and adverse events (*118*); 2 comparative trials (*119*, *120*); n=503; age range 7 mos to 12 yrs]. Only 1 study included children <2 yrs (*121*).	All studies showed efficacy by parasitological assessment of stool samples. Cure rates ranged from 80% to 97%.	Adverse events mild, transient and did not require cessation of treatment. Reported side-effects included anorexia, nausea, vomiting, malaise, and metallic taste.	15 mg/kg in 3 divided doses for 7 days. 20 mg/kg/day for 5 days. 30 mg/kg bd for 7 days.	Oral. No other information provided.
Diloxanide	2 studies [1 comparative trial (*121*): n=39; age range 7 mos to 10 yrs; 1 retrospective study (*122*): n=4371; treatment courses from 1977 to 1990].	Unable to determine efficacy data from information reported in comparative trial.	Most commonly reported side-effect: flatulence. Fewer adverse events reported in those aged 20 mos to 10 yrs than those aged >10 yrs.	25 mg/kg od for 10 days.	Oral. No other information provided.
Pentamidine	3 studies [1 clinical study (*123*), 1 phase II clinical trial (*124*), 1 retrospective study (*125*); n=3133; age range 0 to >15 yrs].	Not reported.	No serious adverse events reported.	4 mg/kg IM once daily for 7 days.	IM injection.
Suramin	No	x	x	x	x

continues

Table 2 *continued*

Drug name(s)	Studies reporting data for children	Efficacy data	Safety data	Doses reported	Formulation(s) reported
Melarsoprol	4 studies [2 RCTs (*126*, *127*), 1 phase II clinical trial (*124*), 1 retrospective analysis (*125*); n=3035; age range 0 to 62 yrs]. All studies included both adults and children.	Melarsoprol+ eflornithine not as effective as nifurtimox+ eflornithine (cure rates 44% vs 94%, respectively).	Significantly toxic. Some deaths attributable to complications of treatment. Poorly tolerated by all age groups. Very young (<2 yrs) more prone to jaundice and rash than adults. Lower incidence of encephalopathic syndrome in preschool-age children, but higher mortality rate in those that did develop it.	Over 26 days: 3 series of 4 daily IV infusions starting at 1.2 mg/kg, increasing to 3.6 mg/kg with a 7 day interval between series. 1.8 mg/kg/day for 10 days. 2.2 mg/kg/day for 10 days.	IV infusion.
Eflornithine	5 studies [3 RCTs (*126*, *128*, *129*), 1 retrospective study (*125*), 1 clinical trial (*130*); n=3509; age range 0 to 77 yrs]. 2 studies included children <2 yrs (*125*, *130*).	Eflornithine has equal efficacy to melarsoprol.	Number of adverse events increased with longer duration of treatment, but only statistically significant for diarrhoea and infections. Less toxic than melarsoprol.	100 mg/kg every 6 hours for either 7 or 14 days. 200 mg/kg every 12 hours for 14 days. 100 mg/kg IV every 6 hours for 14 days, followed by 75 mg/kg orally every 6 hours for 21 days.	Oral. IV infusion.

continues

Table 2 *continued*

Drug name(s)	Studies reporting data for children	Efficacy data	Safety data	Doses reported	Formulation(s) reported
Benznidazole	7 studies [4 RCTs (*131–134*), 1 follow-up study (*135*), 1 observational study (*136*), 1 control programme study (*137*) (MSF project); n= 3400; age range newborn to 18 yrs].	3 studies (*131–133*) showed efficacy in comparison to placebo in children with indeterminate or early stage *T. cruzi*.	Minor adverse events (gastrointestinal disorders; rash). No deaths reported.	2.5 mg/kg bd for 60 days. 5 mg/kg/day 7.5 g/kg once daily for 30 or 60 days. 7.5 mg/kg bd or tds for 60 days. Maximum dose 300 mg/day.	100-mg tablets ground up, and capsules filled with 8, 10, 13, and 15 mg powder to treat neonates according to weight.
Nifurtimox (N)	2 studies [2 RCTs (*126, 129*); n >54; age range 5 yrs to 62 yrs]. Not possible to extract paediatric specific data from either study.	Only used in combination with eflornithine (E) or melarsoprol (M). N+E more effective than M+E (cure rates 94% vs 44%, respectively).	Combination of N+E well tolerated. Low fatality rate compared to melarsoprol (0.76% vs 6%).	15 mg/kg/day in divided doses; 8 hourly for 10 days. 20 mg/kg/d 8 hourly for 10 days.	Oral.

[a] **Abbreviations used in table:**
RCT = randomized controlled trial; mos = months; yrs = years; tds = 3 times daily; od = once daily; bd = twice daily; mf = microfilarial load; d = day.

Section 6.2: Antibacterial medicines

Fluoroquinolones (review) – Children

The Committee had requested a review of quinolones with a focus on safety in children. The current EMLc includes ciprofloxacin (without a square box). Ciprofloxacin is listed in the EML with a square box and ofloxacin as an antituberculosis medicine on the Complementary List, with levofloxacin as an alternative. The review was prepared by Dr Jennifer A Goldman and Dr Gregory L Kearns.

The review conclusions were supported by Dr Mario Raviglione, Director of the Stop TB Department, WHO. Expert reviews were prepared by Professor Noël Cranswick and Professor Anita Zaidi.

The Committee noted that quinolones have been available since the 1960s but findings in juvenile beagle dogs of joint cartilage and tendons alterations, associated with evidence of tendonitis and tendon ruptures in adults, stopped the development for children. Despite these findings, favourable characteristics of quinolones (in terms of pharmacokinetics, possible oral route, and spectrum of activity) resulted in a progressive introduction into paediatric treatment.

The Committee considered efficacy data in cystic fibrosis and in gastrointestinal infections (multidrug-resistant salmonellosis/typhoid fever and shigellosis) as summarized in the review by Algasham & Nahata (*138*) (see review Tables 2 and 3). Data from 4 trials in cystic fibrosis and 12 in GI infections show high cure rates with various fluoroquinolones. The Committee noted that there are reports of efficacy in other serious conditions such as meningitis in children and TB.

The Committee considered available safety data, as presented in the review, and additional data identified by the Secretariat. In children, the Committee noted that there is no large prospective randomized trial assessing safety of fluoroquinolones, but three retrospective analyses of joint safety in children were identified. Two reviews (*139*, *140*) were performed by Johnson & Johnson, manufacturer of levofloxacin. There was one independent study: a cohort study, comparing 276 children receiving fluoroquinolones with 246 controls receiving other antibacterial medicines. In the quinolone group, there were more adverse events, all transient, and no persistent musculoskeletal lesions were observed. Among fluoroquinolones, pefloxacin had higher incidence compared to ciprofloxacin (18.2% versus 3.3%, respectively) (*141*).

Levofloxacin safety data from three large trials including 2523 children were reviewed by Noel GJ et al. (*140*). There were more spontaneous reports of musculoskeletal events (mostly arthralgias) with levofloxacin than other antibiotics (2.1% versus 0.9%; $P = 0.04$). Five patients had either CT or MRI investigations, but no joint damage could be identified. The Secretariat identified a randomized trial of ciprofloxacin that reported safety data from 335 children (mean age 6.3 years) treated with ciprofloxacin compared with 349 children treated with unspecified comparators. This study reported an incidence of suspected drug-related arthropathy, based on clinical signs and symptoms by day 42, of 7.2% and 4.6%. At one year, the incidence of drug-related arthropathy was 9.0% and 5.7%, not statistically significant.

The Committee noted that other adverse effects reported with fluoroquinolones include phototoxicity, prolonged QT interval, acute liver failure (which led to trovafloxacin withdrawal from the market), convulsions (in particular in combination with NSAIDs), and risk of haemolysis in patients with glucose-6-phosphate dehydrogenase (G6PD) deficiency.

The Committee concluded that the effectiveness and safety of fluoroquinolones in the treatment of serious bacterial infections in children have been sufficiently established. Taking into consideration the desirable pharmacokinetic (PK) characteristics and antibacterial spectrum of the class, the Committee considered that there was enough evidence supporting the use in children, in life-threatening conditions such as resistant TB, dysentery, and cholera. In resource-poor countries, the Committee considered that the oral route of administration was a substantial advantage and cost effective. The development of antibiotic resistance will be an issue, should wider use occur. There should be careful restriction of the use of fluoroquinolones to prevent the development of resistance.

The Committee therefore retained ciprofloxacin on the EMLc, but did not recommend the addition of a square box to the current listing.

Section 8: Antineoplastic agents, immunosuppressives and medicines used in palliative care (review) – Children

In 2007, when the first EMLc was published, the Expert Committee noted that immunosuppressives and cytotoxics are essential for treating tumours in children, but requested a review of the medicines listed to ensure that they are appropriate for the treatment of common tumours in children. A review was prepared by Dr Ronald Barr and Dr Paul Rogers, Children's & Women's Health Centre of British Columbia Branch, Canada.

Expert reviews were prepared by Dr Lenita Wannmacher and Dr Kalle Hoppu.

The most common paediatric malignancies are leukaemias (30%), brain or other nervous system cancers (22.3%), neuroblastoma (7.3%), Wilms tumours (5.6%), and non-Hodgkin lymphoma (4.5%), but there are regional variations, e.g. retinoblastoma is frequent in parts of India and Burkitt lymphoma in numerous countries of sub-Saharan Africa. While these diseases may be less frequent than tumours in adults, treatment of paediatric tumours have high rates of success.

Access to high-level supportive care, diagnostic techniques, combinations of anti-infectives, intensive care, and specialized expertise is a necessary condition for the treatment of paediatric malignancies, but has important cost and resources consequences.

In all settings, successes in the treatment of neoplastic conditions in both adults and children have depended on the use of treatment protocols, rather than the use of individual medicines. The Committee endorsed the recommendation that, for the Essential Medicines List, medicines selected for the treatment of paediatric oncology conditions should be (1) aimed at common treatable tumours in childhood and (2) based on a protocol approach to optimize efficacy and to avoid unacceptably high rates of treatment-related morbidity and mortality (*142*). The review prioritized three common and treatable conditions: acute lymphoblastic leukaemia (ALL), Wilms tumour (WT, or nephroblastoma), and Burkitt lymphoma (BL), and proposed a stepwise approach to the availability of essential medicines. This was agreed by the Committee and the discussion below reflects the decision to include the medicines necessary for steps 1 and 2, as listed in the review. Step 1 designates a common protocol for all patients; step 2 introduces additional drugs for high-risk patients; step 3 includes dose intensification and the need for alternative forms of medicine in steps 1 and 2 (e.g. asparaginase); step 4 include medicines requiring intensive monitoring and supportive treatment to ensure safe use (e.g. high dose methotrexate requiring 'rescue'); and step 5 covers the full range of treatment options including transplant where appropriate.

Acute lymphoblastic leukaemia

The Committee reviewed the treatment of ALL based on three principles: (1) the need to maintain long-term treatment (about 5 years); (2) the need to prevent drug resistance; and (3) the fact that the CNS and testes require special treatment to avoid relapses. Radiotherapy was widely used for this, but is now increasingly restricted.

Clinical trials in ALL performed by major study groups (*143*) form the evidence that led to improved outcomes of children with ALL and cure rates of over 80% in developed countries. Prediction of treatment response can be assessed by administration of prednisone before induction. Prednisone is not on the EMLc but the Committee considered that prednisolone has similar therapeutic use.

The Committee considered and agreed to the proposal made in the review for a stepwise approach to essential drug requirements, allowing increasing treatment requirements as experience of management of patients with increasing risk factors is progressively acquired (see Table 3). The Committee considered that medicines listed in steps 1 and 2 should all be on

Table 3
Stepwise approach to essential drug requirements

Steps	Medicines
1: A common protocol for all patients	Prednisolone (oral), methylprednisolone (IV), dexamethasone (oral), vincristine (IV), asparaginase (IM), MTX (IM, IT, and oral), and mercaptopurine (oral)
2: Additional drugs for high-risk patients	Doxorubicin (IV), daunorubicin (IV), cyclophosphamide (IV), cytosine arabinoside (IV and IT), hydrocortisone (IT), MTX (IV) at doses not requiring 'rescue', and thioguanine (PO)
3: Dose intensification and need for alternate forms of medicine in steps 1 and 2	Other forms of asparaginase
4: Medicines requiring intensive monitoring and supportive treatment to ensure safe use	High doses of methotrexate with rescue leucovorin/folinic acid (PO and IV)
5: The full range of treatment options including transplant where appropriate	Haematopoietic stem cell transplantation at a high level of care; step 5 requires availability of busulfan (PO and IV), cyclosporin (PO and IV), etoposide (PO and IV), thioguanine (PO), and imatinib

IT: intrathecal; PO: by mouth; IV: intravenous; IM: intramuscular.

the Complementary List, so recommended the inclusion of methylprednisolone and thioguanine in addition to those already listed. The Committee decided not to add further medicines to the EMLc but highlighted the value of the progress approach to developing systems to provide treatment of ALL in children.

Lymphomas including Burkitt lymphoma

BL accounts for 40–50% of lymphoma cases in malaria non-endemic areas but approximately 80% in endemic areas. In Africa, BL may account for up to 45% of childhood cancer. CNS involvement at diagnosis is considered the strongest risk factor for relapse, requiring more intensive treatment.

The core three medicines for the treatment of BL are cyclophosphamide (IV, PO), methotrexate (oral) and vincristine (IV), allowing survival rates of 25% and 33% in Uganda and Ghana. Further studies showed that the addition of prednisone, escalation of doses of methotrexate, and dose intensity had beneficial effects. Intensive protocols aimed at B cell non-Hodgkin lymphoma and B cell ALL, including also etoposide, doxorubicin and cytarabine, have led to 90% event-free survival in developed countries (e.g. protocol LMB89) (*144*); and these protocols have been adapted to low-income countries. A recent report from 4 African countries showed a 1-year survival of 68% with 6 cycles of a combination of methotrexate, cyclophosphamide and vincristine. An adaptation of LMB89 in Malawi using methotrexate, cyclophosphamide, prednisone and vincristine resulted in acceptable toxicity and 50% event-free survival, at low cost (*145*). However, the Committee noted that access to adequate supportive care is necessary for intensive treatment in particular.

Typically the treatment includes three phases. Induction requires cyclophosphamide, prednisone and vincristine, to minimize the risk of tumour lysis syndrome. Intensive chemotherapy after induction requires the above with doxorubicin, and methotrexate with leucovorin rescue. Consolidation requires cytarabine and methotrexate, and cytarabine with etoposide.

The Committee concluded that all medicines mentioned above are included in the EMLc (Complementary List). For tumour lysis syndrome, allopurinol is included but not urate oxidase.

Wilms tumour (nephroblastoma)

WTs have an incidence of 10, 8, and 4 per million in Black, Caucasian, and Asian populations, respectively.

The Committee considered that high-quality RCTs support the current treatment of WT. The Committee noted that initial staging and histology are established by initial surgery, except when tumour rupture or extensive venous invasion have occurred and initial chemotherapy is required. Abdominal radiation therapy may be combined with chemotherapy, with lung irradiation in cases of metastases.

Actinomycin D (dactinomycin) remains an essential component of treatment.

The Committee noted that in lower risk WTs, dactinomycin, vincristine, and doxorubicin are used, with 90% survival rates reported in developed countries. For higher-risk WTs, cyclophosphamide and more recently ifosfamide, carboplatin, and etoposide are added. A combination of ifosfamide, carboplatin, and etoposide is used in some relapses. For bilateral tumours, preoperative chemotherapy with dactinomycin and vincristine is used, and surgery aims to preserve the function of the less affected kidney.

In low-income countries, the survival rate is much lower due to a combination of late referrals (advanced massive tumours), and lack of surgery, radiation oncology, and pathology expertise (*146*). Preoperative chemotherapy (dactinomycin and vincristine) is favoured as it allows correcting malnutrition and infections before surgery (*147*).

All the medicines required above, except ifosfamide, are already included in the EMLc.

The Committee recommended deleting chlorambucil, 5-fluorouracil, bleomycin, dacarbazine, procarbazine, ifosfamide, and etoposide from the EMLc, as they did not appear in steps 1 and 2 of the protocols for the three priority conditions. The WHO Model Formulary needs to clearly identify appropriate protocols for the use of the medicines included in the List.

Adjunctive treatments

Among adjuvant medicines, the Committee reviewed urate oxidase, 2-mercapto ethane sulfonate sodium (MESNa), glutamic acid, granulocyte colony-stimulating factor (G-CSF), and granulocyte macrophage colony-stimulating factor (GM-CSF), in the light of the decision to support inclusion of step 1 and 2 medicines for the three priority conditions.

The Committee evaluated a Cochrane Review of five studies (including 336 treated children) in the prevention and treatment of tumour lysis syndrome, which concluded that urate oxidase is highly effective in reducing serum uric acid. One RCT, with three case–control studies of low quality, comparing urate oxidase and allopurinol showed no significant difference in mortality or renal failure. The Committee did not recommend that urate oxidase be included in the EML, but decided to list allopurinol as an adjunctive treatment.

MESNa is used to correct high-dose cyclophosphamide-induced haemorrhagic cystitis or haematuria. Toxicity increases with the (total) dose and is more frequent in children aged less than 5 years. The Committee noted that MESNa had been added to the main EML in 2009 and therefore recommended its inclusion on the EMLc, listed as a medicine for adjunctive treatment.

Section 8.2: Cytotoxic medicines

Imatinib (inclusion) – Children and adolescents

A review of the use of imatinib in children with chronic myelogenous leukaemia (CML) was prepared by Dr Ronald D Barr, Department of Pediatrics, Pathology and Medicine, McMaster University at the request of the Secretariat for the Expert Committee on the Selection and Use of Essential Medicines.

Expert reviews of the application were prepared by Professor Noël Cranswick and Dr Gregory L Kearns. Comments were received from Dr Shanti Mendis, Coordinator, WHO Department of Chronic Diseases Prevention and Management.

The Committee noted the rarity of CML in children, the limited evidence of efficacy and long-term safety in children, and the high cost of the medicine, and therefore recommended that imatinib should not be added to the EMLc.

Finally, the Committee recommended that Section 8.3 Hormones and antihormones be deleted, as the medicines previously included were to be listed under each priority condition.

Section 8.4: Medicines used in palliative care

The medicines listed in Section 8.4, medicines used in palliative care, had been comprehensively updated in 2009. The Committee confirmed that this section should include a comprehensive list of medicines for palliative care, as advocacy in this area is still needed. The Committee recommended that the following amendments be made:

- deleting the restriction of use of ibuprofen for bone pain, in line with the recent WHO guideline on persisting pain (*148*);
- adding ondansetron, which is already on the EMLc;
- adding fluoxetine, which is already on the EMLc for the treatment of depression; and
- adding midazolam, also considered at this meeting, for use in procedures in children.

A recent Cochrane meta-analysis (10 RCTs) found that polyethylene glycol was better than lactulose in both adults and children, except for relief of abdominal pain (*149*). The Committee noted that despite guideline recommendations for the use of senna or docusate sodium, no trial supporting their use could be identified (*150*). Noting the lack of available evidence, the Committee recommended addition of lactulose to this section.

The Committee also expressed the need to complete an evidence-based review of the listing of medicines for palliative care in adults.

Section 10: Medicines affecting the blood

Section 10.2: Medicines affecting coagulation

Antithrombotic (review) – Children

A review of antithrombotic medicines used in children was submitted by Dr F Newall (Melbourne, Australia).

Expert reviews were provided by Dr Kalle Hoppu and Dr Gregory L Kearns. The current EMLc includes phytometadione, and on the Complementary List, heparin sodium, protamine sulfate (antidote) and warfarin □.

The public health relevance of thrombotic disorders in children was considered. Venous thromboembolism may occur in children, in particular related to central venous access and more rarely malignancies, vascular malformations, trauma, and surgery. The reported incidence in Canadian children was 5.3–8 per 10 000 but only one publication relating to developing countries was identified without incidence data. Arterial thromboembolism is unlikely in children. Predisposing factors include intra-arterial devices, arterial malformations, surgery, and congenital heart diseases (with possible arterial ischaemic stroke).

The Committee reviewed the evidence available for unfractionated heparin, low molecular weight heparin (LMWH), acenocoumarol, and warfarin.

The evidence of effectiveness and safety included 20 studies in children but only four RCTs. Studies included 10 to 366 individuals, aged from birth to more than 19 years in prevention or treatment of arterial or venous thromboembolic events. Doses varied from 10 IU/kg per hr to 500 IU/kg per day, with or without loading doses. One RCT concluded that heparin was more effective than placebo in preventing cool pulse-less extremities in cardiac angiography (*151*). One RCT showed that individualized doses were more effective than standard doses in preventing blood loss and the need for transfusion (*152*). Another RCT compared unfractionated heparin, LMWH, and vitamin K antagonists in children and reported a 12.5% rate of major bleeding in the UF heparin/vitamin K antagonists arm compared to 5.65% in the LMWH group (*153*). During cardiopulmonary bypass, children received more heparin when titration was individualized (*154*).

In paediatric populations, normal ranges for laboratory parameters for monitoring use of unfractionated heparin are unknown. There are three methods: protamine titration, anti-Xa and activated partial thromboplastin time (APTT). APTT levels are increased in children compared to adults. A protamine titration assay range of 0.2 to 0.4 units/ml or anti-Xa range of 0.35 to 0.7 units/ml results in a 3- or 4-fold increase in APTT prolongation over that observed in adults.

Adverse effects of unfractionated heparins are dominated by bleeding, as shown by Massicote et al. (*153*). Heparin-induced thrombocytopaenia occurs in less than 3% of adult patients exposed for five days or more; observations may indicate a lower risk in children (*155*). Accidental overdose is a significant risk due to different concentrations (factor 10 or 100) and the need for dilution. The Committee concluded that unfractionated heparin was effective and required monitoring for safe use. It therefore recommended that unfractionated heparin be retained on the EMLc Complementary List.

Vitamin K antagonists include warfarin, phencoproumon, and acenocoumarol. Few cohort studies of use in children were identified: six prospective and two retrospective studies on warfarin, and one prospective and one retrospective on acenocoumarol. Patient populations on warfarin ranged from 15 to 319 and children's ages from less than 1 year to more than 19 years for the treatment or secondary prevention of very diverse conditions, e.g. deep venous thrombosis or congenital heart disease. Mean warfarin doses ranged from 0.07 mg/kg to 0.33 mg/kg. Acenocoumarol was used in similar conditions in children aged 2 months to 18 years at mean dose ranges of 0.06 mg/kg to 0.2 mg/kg or 2 mg per day.

Monitoring of warfarin or acenocoumarol is based on prothrombin time, expressed as international normalized ratio (INR). In children monitoring should be based on venous INR or better, capillary INR. Bleeding rates in children were estimated at 20% for minor events per patient year, and 1.7–3.2% for major events depending on therapy intensity (*156*). Warfarin may have effects on bone mineral density as vitamin K is necessary to bone growth, but no prospective data exist in children and data in adults are conflicting.

The Committee recommended that warfarin be retained with a square box, as acenocoumarol may be an effective alternative in children.

LMWHs are currently not authorized for use in children by stringent authorities. Eight publications were identified on the use of LMWH in children, including two RCTs using reviparin. Studies included populations ranging from 24 to 186 children aged 0 to 18 years. Doses could not be compared as they were expressed in units, or mg/kg. Dose response was less predictable in children than in adults. A RCT compared unfractionated heparin and Vitamin K antagonist with LMWH in 76 children with venous thromboembolism. At 3 months, there were less recurrent venous thromboembolism or death in the LMWH treated group and fewer major bleeds (*153*). The second trial in children receiving central venous lines was terminated prematurely due to slow accrual and was underpowered. There was no significant difference in central venous line-related thrombosis between LMWH and placebo. One patient had a major bleed and there were two deaths in the standard care group (*157*). The Committee concluded that effectiveness of LMWH in children is insufficiently demonstrated, and the risks seem comparable to unfractionated heparin and vitamin K antagonists. In addition the Committee considered that LMWH requires monitoring by anti-Xa assays, which is costly. They are more expensive than unfractionated heparin and the monitoring is also more expensive. The Committee recommended not to include LMWH in the EMLc.

The Committee invited an application for the inclusion of LMWH or alternatives in adults.

Section 15: Disinfectants and antiseptics

Chlorhexidine (change of formulation) – Children

In 2009, an application was considered by the Committee for an additional strength of chlorhexidine, for use in umbilical cord care, to prevent neonatal sepsis. At that time the Committee noted that there was no commercially available product in the specific strength used in the trial, and, as the existing formulation (20%) could be diluted to the trial product strength, the EMLc was not amended.

An updated application has been submitted by the Program for Appropriate Technology in Health (PATH), to replace the 20% chlorhexidine, which requires dilution, with a ready-made 7.1% chlorhexidine digluconate solution and gel. The application was supported by a company developing such a formulation (Popular, Bangladesh) and Research Training and Management (RTM) International, from Bangladesh. Expert reviews were prepared by Professor David Ofori-Adjei and Mr Andy Gray.

The current EML includes topical chlorhexidine 5% and 20% as digluconate. Chlorhexidine is registered by stringent regulatory authorities at other concentrations and in other indications.

The importance of omphalitis as a cause of neonatal mortality is well established. Infections account for an estimated 1.44 million deaths, and about half of deaths in regions with high neonatal mortality rates (*158*). Hygienic delivery and postnatal-care practices are widely promoted as important interventions to reduce risk of omphalitis and death (*159*).

The Committee noted that the evidence for effectiveness of chlorhexidine in cord care in the context of developing countries was reviewed in 2008. An additional trial was presented in this application, a randomized controlled non-inferiority comparison between a 4% gel and aqueous solution that showed non-inferiority between the two presentations, based on a biomarker. The Committee noted that two more cluster-randomized controlled trials are ongoing but not yet reported in the literature (Arifeen et al. 2010; Bhutta et al. 2010; *160*). There are no reports of toxicity with chlorhexidine use for cord care; while chlorhexidine, similar to other antiseptics, delays cord separation, this is not related to the incidence of omphalitis (*161*).

Information about the costs of the gel and the solution of 4% chlorhexidine was reported in a trial from 2010 (*158*). The cost of single swabbing was estimated to be the same price (US$ 0.02) for the gel as for the aqueous solution, based on a preparation by a company in Nepal.

The problem remains that, as in 2009, a commercially available preparation of 7.1% chlorhexidine digluconate solution or gel (delivering 4% chlorhexidine) is not yet available. While the 20% requires dilution and manipulation and is clearly not optimal, until there is a commercially available product of the strength and formulation used in the trials, the current listing cannot be amended. However, the Committee noted that an optimized 4% chlorhexidine is listed as one of the priority products for development by WHO on the Priority Medicines list for maternal and child health and therefore flagged it as a 'missing' essential medicine, given the impact on mortality suggested in the trials.

Section 16: Diuretics

Mannitol (review) – Children

In October 2007, the Subcommittee of the Expert Committee for the Selection and Use of Essential Medicines requested that the role of Mannitol in children be reviewed in light of potentially newer and more effective medicines. A systematic review of the role of mannitol in the therapy of children was prepared by Dr Fatemeh Tavakkoli, Pharm. D Candidate, University of Maryland School of Pharmacy, Maryland, USA.

Expert reviews were prepared by Professor Jennifer Welbeck and Dr Kalle Hoppu.

The Committee noted that the review provided a comprehensive summary of the available evidence for the use of mannitol in the treatment of cerebral oedema, diabetic ketoacidosis, asthma, and cystic fibrosis in children. The Committee noted that raised intracranial pressure (ICP) is a common and serious consequence of traumatic brain injury (TBI) and also a frequent and life-threatening complication of diabetic ketoacidosis (DKA) in children.

The Committee noted the paucity of high-quality RCTs comparing mannitol with placebo or other hyperosmolar agents to support the safety and efficacy of mannitol for the management of raised ICP secondary to TBI, DKA, and malaria in paediatric patients. They also noted that there are few data to validate different regimens of mannitol administration. However, the Committee noted that there is some evidence from observational studies in children that have shown clinical improvement following the use of mannitol for the management of raised ICP secondary to TBI or DKA (*162–164*). There was no evidence to support its use in the management of raised ICP secondary to cerebral malaria.

Due to the fact that raised ICP secondary to traumatic brain injury or DKA have serious health consequences in children and mannitol has been used in both adults and children for the treatment of raised ICP with evidence of clinical improvement, and there is limited evidence to recommend a suitable alternative at this time, the Committee recommended that mannitol be maintained on the EMLc until evidence supporting a suitable alternative treatment becomes available.

Spironolactone (review) – Children

In October 2007, the Subcommittee of the Expert Committee for the Selection and Use of Essential Medicines requested that the role of spironolactone in children be reviewed in light of potentially newer and more effective medicines. A systematic review of the role of spironolactone in the therapy of children was prepared by Dr Fatemeh Tavakkoli, Pharm. D Candidate, University of Maryland School of Pharmacy, Maryland, USA.

An expert review was prepared by Professor Noël Cranswick.

The Committee noted that the review provided a comprehensive summary of the available evidence for the use of spironolactone in the treatment of congestive heart failure, hyperaldosteronism, Bartter syndrome, precocious puberty, Alport syndrome, hypertrichosis, bronchodysplasia, syndrome of apparent mineralocorticoid excess, and nephrotic syndrome in children.

The Committee noted the paucity of high-quality RCTs comparing spironolactone with placebo or other appropriate therapeutic interventions to support the safety and efficacy of spironolactone in the management of the identified indications in children. The Committee noted there are limited data to validate different regimens of administration of spironolactone. The Committee commented that there is a new selective aldosterone receptor antagonist, eplerenone, that has recently been approved for the management of heart failure, but it is not currently recommended for children and no evidence to support its efficacy and safety were presented in the review. The Committee recommended that spironolactone be maintained on the EMLc, on the Complementary List.

Section 17: Gastrointestinal medicines

Section 17.5: Medicines used in diarrhoea

Section 17.5.2: Medicines for diarrhoea in children

Zinc sulfate (new formulation) – Children

The Department of Child and Adolescent Health, WHO submitted a proposal to include a 20-mg oral dosage form of zinc sulfate, to match available products and for cost reasons. Zinc sulfate is currently listed on the EML as:

Oral liquid: in 10 mg per unit dosage forms.
Tablet: in 10 mg per unit dosage forms.

Expert reviews were provided by Mr Andy Gray and Professor David Ofori-Adjei.

The Committee noted that when zinc sulfate was originally added to the EML in 2005, only the 10-mg dosage was listed. No commercial products were then available and the basis for the listing was to ensure that 20-mg scored tablets should not be cut in half for use in infants aged less than 6 months, as this practice could not ensure that the dose of zinc administered to these infants would be precise enough. In 2010, more than 40 manufacturers are producing zinc tablets for use in the management of diarrhoea as 20-mg zinc tablets in order to reduce the cost of zinc treatment for children aged more than 6 months. Supplementing children with two 10-mg zinc tablets costs twice as much as supplementation with one single 20-mg zinc tablet. Keeping the cost of treatment as low as possible is essential to increase access to, and coverage of, the treatment.

Two publications were submitted (*165, 166*) in support of supplementation and several additional publications were identified by the Secretariat. The main issue considered by the Committee was the safety and palatability of a 20-mg dose form for children aged less than 6 months.

There is conflicting evidence on the efficacy of zinc in the subgroup of infants aged less than 6 months. A Cochrane Review stratified by age included 18 trials (13 in acute diarrhoea), of which two trials were in 1334 infants aged less than 6 months (*165, 167*). The review concluded that zinc reduced diarrhoea duration measured at day 3, 5, and 7 but there was significant heterogeneity. In the Cochrane Review of zinc (*168*) three more trials used doses higher than the currently recommended 10 mg and included some infants aged less than 6 months. The combined analysis of vomiting in trials of all infants aged less than 6 months and above, showed an increased risk of vomiting (RR 2.01; 95% CI 1.06–3.81, 1505 children, three trials). In these three trials infants received 20-mg zinc sulfate tablet (*169*), 15 mg zinc (*170*), and 20-mg zinc sulfate solution (*171*), respectively. The actual number of infants aged less than 6 months was not specified.

The Committee considered that zinc safety is not a major issue, even given at 20 mg in infants aged less than 6 months. Zinc administration is associated with a single reported adverse effect, vomiting, but there is no clear dose–effect relationship. Vomiting is generally limited to a single episode after the first dose in the vast majority of children. It was decided to list the flexible, dispersible 20-mg oral solid dosage form only. A palatable formulation, which could reduce the risk of vomiting, would be necessary. The Committee noted that appropriate oral liquid forms are not widely available and therefore decided to delete this dosage form.

Section 18: Hormones

Section 18.5: Insulins and other antidiabetic agents

Review of the use of oral hypoglycaemic agents in children (review) – Children

In 2009, the Subcommittee on Selection and Use of Essential Medicines for children requested a review of the efficacy and safety of the use of oral antidiabetic medicines in children. A review was prepared by Mr Alfred Sakeyfio and expert reviews were provided by Professor Noël Cranswick and Dr Lenita Wannmacher. The products currently on the EML are metformin 500-mg tablets and glibenclamide 2.5-mg and 5-mg tablets. Metformin is listed on the Complementary List of the EMLc.

The review identified a limited number of systematic reviews and small randomized trials in children that evaluate the effects of different oral hypoglycaemic medicines. The populations in the trials were children aged six to 18 years, mostly in studies in high- and middle-income settings. Doses of drugs used in studies were not clearly described. Sample sizes were small, most of the studies were relatively short-term, and outcomes measured were surrogate markers, usually change in HbA1c. This outcome has not been validated as a surrogate in diabetes in children.

Based on a systematic review (*172*) metformin is suggested to be potentially useful in children aged more than 8 years. The number of studies included in the systematic review is not stated; the total number of patients included was 142. The review also briefly covers other evidence for other oral hypoglycaemics – acarbose, pramlintide, sitagliptin, repaglinide, mitiglinide, pioglitazone – but provides only limited evidence about comparative safety of these medicines in children and no information about comparative costs.

The Committee noted that metformin is licensed by the US Food and Drug Administration and several European countries for use in children aged 10–16 years. Glibenclamide is not licensed for use in children.

The Committee decided to retain metformin on the Complementary List of the EMLc, but not add any other oral hypoglycaemic medicines until there is further evidence of their efficacy and safety in children. Countries facing increasing disease burdens from diabetes should be cautious about increasing access to oral hypoglycaemics other than metformin, as the evidence to support their use in paediatric patients is lacking.

The Committee also requested a review of the comparative safety of different sulfonylureas in elderly patients.

6. Applications for the 17th Model List and the 3rd EMLc

Section 1: Anaesthetics

Following suggestions concerning the listing of different inhalational anaesthetic medicines, a review of Section 1 and Section 20 of the EML was prepared by Dr Tim Robertson (University of Newcastle, Australia) and Dr Anna Louise Ridge (WHO Department of Essential Medicines and Pharmaceutical Policies) to allow the Committee to update the section. The proposals were:

(1) add isoflurane (as a cost-effective alternative to halothane), propofol (for both induction and maintenance of anaesthesia), midazolam (more effective than promethazine or diazepam for sedation), and atracurium (superior to alcuronium); and

(2) delete thiopental, diazepam, promethazine (less effective than midazolam), and alcuronium.

Expert reviews were provided by Professor Abdol Majid Cheraghali and Dr Gregory L Kearns. Comments were received from Médecins Sans Frontières supporting the review, but proposing retention of thiopental as a useful and cost-effective alternative to propofol.

The Committee noted that in the developing world anaesthesia is often delivered by non-medical staff or medical staff with limited training and resources with respect to facilities and equipment.

The Committee reviewed the evidence on inhalational anaesthetics.

Currently halothane (square box) and nitrous oxide are the only inhalational anaesthetics on the EML. Halothane is widely used in both induction and maintenance, in adults and children but has been gradually replaced in developed countries by isoflurane, enflurane, desflurane, and sevoflurane for safety reasons. Ensuring availability of halothane is increasingly problematic in many settings. None of these medicines is best in all situations and the choice is determined by the availability of the medicines and specific vaporizers.

While isoflurane causes less hepatic failure than halothane (*173*), and has advantages for maintenance, it is unsuitable for induction. Enflurane also has a lower rate of hepatic failure and less cardiovascular toxicity than halothane, but increases the risk of seizure, and has to be avoided in patients with epilepsy. Isoflurane and enflurane have more rapid onset and recovery times than halothane. Sevoflurane and desflurane have the most rapid onset and offset of action and few adverse effects, such as airways irritation for desflurane (*174*), agitation in more than 20% of children during recovery, and convulsions with sevoflurane. Both sevoflurane and desflurane are more expensive than halothane, isoflurane, or enflurane.

The Committee decided to include isoflurane but not enflurane (due to the risks of convulsions) or sevoflurane (due to cost). Halothane should remain, but without a square box, as this would not be listed as the examplar of all inhalation agents. Where available, halothane provides an affordable option for induction and maintenance. However, where availability is an issue, isoflurane provides an acceptable option for maintenance. The Committee also decided to divide this section between injectable and inhalational agents (and oxygen).

The Committee noted that nitrous oxide can be used as a single agent where general anaesthesia is not required, or in combination with inhalational anaesthetics. Use in combination reduces the dose, toxicity, and costs of inhalational drugs. The Committee therefore decided to retain nitrous oxide in the EML.

The Committee reviewed the evidence on IV anaesthetics. Ketamine and thiopental (☐) are on the current EML. A comparison of IV anaesthetics was provided in the application (Table 5).

Ketamine is the most widely used in developing countries. It has few effects on the cardiovascular system, and although apnoea can occur after injection, airways reflexes are preserved and respiratory depression does not occur. Ketamine is associated with hallucinations and vivid dreams at recovery (*175*).

The Committee considered that thiopental, propofol, and etomidate have been shown to be safe induction agents (*176*). For thiopental, repeat dosing can induce prolonged somnolence and has a hang-over effect. The Committee noted that there is conflicting information on different haemodynamic effects of propofol and thiopental. A 2001 systematic review concluded that there were no differences in safety and efficacy between propofol and thiopental based on evidence obtained in stable patients in non-emergency department settings (*177*). While etomidate has possible advantages for use in patients in shock – as it does not produce cardiovascular depression (*176*) – it is associated with adrenal suppression even after single use, which limits its use. Etomidate was therefore not added to the EML.

The Committee was of the opinion that thiopental could be deleted due to its safety profile and predictable difficulties in supply in the future, but that it needed to be retained as an alternative to propofol.

Preoperative medications and sedation for short-term procedures

The Committee reviewed the medicines used preoperatively and those for sedation for short-term procedures.

The review suggested that midazolam may be as safe as, but more effective than, diazepam for short-term procedures, due to its short duration of action, and amnesic properties (*175*). Midazolam has better efficacy than promethazine in children in the preoperative setting (*178*). The Committee also considered the separate review of midazolam. The committee concluded that injectable midazolam should be included in the EML to replace diazepam, listed with a □ symbol.

Muscle relaxants (Section 20)

The current EML includes suxamethonium, alcuronium (□), and vecuronium (□). The review proposes to replace alcuronium by atracurium (□).

Alcuronium has a slow onset and long duration of action, with more adverse effects than other non-depolarizing agents (*179*). It is no longer registered by stringent regulatory authorities (United States, United Kingdom, France). Atracurium has fewer adverse effects, although it can cause histamine release. Rocuronium and vecuronium have longer onset of action but decreased risk of tachycardia. Pancuronium has an even longer onset and duration of action. The Committee noted that the information in the review showed that, within the class, atracurium is cheaper than others except pancuronium (Table 7 in the application) and therefore recommended the replacement of alcuronium with atracurium (□), due to its comparative effectiveness and safety profile, current availability, and cost. The Committee recommended that this section (Section 20) be reviewed before the next Expert Committee meeting, to consider which longer-acting agents were needed, and which were specifically useful in children.

Section 1.1: General anaesthetics and oxygen

Ether (re-instatement)

Ether was deleted from the WHO Model List of Essential Medicines in 2005. The WHO Expert Committee cited ether's cumbersome transport and storage requirements, its declining use and the availability of the preferred alternative fluorinated inhalational agent: halothane. At the time, both the International Society of Drug Bulletins (ISDB) and the World Federation of Societies of Anaesthesiologists (WFSA) had suggested that ether be retained on the WHO Model List because of its low cost and relative safety when used by inexperienced staff, and in the absence of oxygen.

The Committee noted a new request is made for re-instatement from the WFSA (Dr Haydn Perndt), supported by Dr Wilson (Pdt, Association of Anaesthetists of Great Britain and Ireland), Dr Dobson (United Kingdom), Dr Coonan, and Dr Paquet (Canada), Dr Sundnes (Norway), Dr Teweldebrhan (Eritrea), Dr Fenton, and Dr Goddia (Malawi), Dr Vreede (East Timor), Dr McDougall (Australia), and Dr Towey (Uganda). The request is based on the effectiveness of ether for anaesthesia (pain, sedation, and relaxation), the long experience of ether in developing countries, its safety when no oxygen is available, or in the hands of untrained personnel.

An expert review was provided by Dr Gregory L Kearns.

The Committee reviewed the conclusions of 2005. At that time it was considered that ether had a less favourable benefit–risk balance than halothane in view of halothane's greater precision in controlling anaesthetic state and overall better safety profile despite the known hepatic toxicity. The new application from the World Federation does not contain any new comparative data; it provides the results of two surveys in Uganda concerning ether use as an example from a low-income country (*180*, *181*).

One survey of 97 "anaesthesia providers" reported results from 91 responses, covering mostly large, and district hospitals. It is estimated there are about 350 anaesthesia providers overall in Uganda. The authors (*180*) found that in Uganda, ether is the "most widely used volatile agent and always available to 68% of the respondents". Despite significant use of ether reported in the survey, the Committee considered that anaesthesia for children appeared to be largely ketamine-based due to a lack of disposable airway equipment such as tracheal tubes, facemasks and breathing circuits. Ether was less available than ketamine: ether was reported as always available in 68% of cases, never in 9%, whereas ketamine was always available in 92%, never in 4%, and halothane always in 38% of cases and never in 39% of cases. The Committee also noted that oxygen was reported as always available in 63% of cases, never in 10% in the same survey.

The Committee considered the data from the second survey performed over 2007–2008 in 14 Ugandan districts. The survey concluded that draw-over anaesthesia with either halothane or ether was used in 26/29 hospitals, and oxygen was supplied in them by an electric oxygen concentrator. All hospitals indicated having a supply of oxygen in operating theatres at all times, although nine hospitals did not have a backup generator for power failures, which are common in Uganda.

The availability of ether vaporizers was not discussed in the application.

The Committee noted the risks of ether, which is highly flammable and explosive and incompatible with diathermy. After careful consideration, the Committee concluded that, despite evidence of continued use in some settings, and noting the many inputs provided, ether should not be re-instated on the EML and that alternatives with better benefit–risk balances should be preferred.

Promethazine (deletion) – Adults and children

In 2009, the Committee requested a review of promethazine in preoperative medication and sedation for short-term procedures (adults and children), following the deletion from the EML and EMLc of promethazine for use in postoperative nausea and vomiting. The review was commissioned by the Secretariat and prepared by Dr J Markic and Dr D Sambujnak (Split, Croatia).

Expert reviews were provided by Mr Andy Gray and Professor Jennifer Welbeck. Comments were received from by Dr Bruce Reidenberg, Assistant

Professor of Pharmacology and Pediatrics, Weill Cornell Medical College, New York.

With respect to use in preoperative medication, the Committee noted that the review identified 17 clinical trials of variable quality, including three (*178*, *182*, *183*) in children and 1 systematic review. Doses (oral) of promethazine ranged between 0.5 mg/kg and 1.2 mg/kg in children. In adults the maximum oral dose was 50 mg; parenteral doses ranged between 0.1 and 1.2 mg/kg (IM/IV), or as fixed doses, between 6.25 and 25 mg (IM/IV).

Outcome measures were anxiety, sedation/drowsiness and stress indicators (sleep, various clinical and biochemical indicators). Nine trials had anxiety as primary end-point but only six included a validated scale. Promethazine was generally no different to active comparators (various benzodiazepines) or less effective than midazolam, and superior to placebo for some, but not all, outcomes.

A systematic review on effectiveness of medicines for dental premedication in children was identified in the Cochrane database (*184*). Sixty-one trials involving 3246 children were reviewed. Only one trial included promethazine (*178*); it is reported above and concluded in favour of midazolam over promethazine.

The application reviewed the safety data available in trials. Ten trials reported adverse effects, six in adults including 217 adult subjects exposed to promethazine. In addition to sedation, dry mouth, urinary retention, dizziness, headache, hypotension pruritus, and akathisia were reported. Two further trials in women reported prolonged sedation, nausea, dizziness, dyskinesia, depression, aggression, confusion, diplopia, hallucinations, and heartburn. Two trials in children reported on safety. In the first one, adverse effects were reported in 37% of 40 patients treated with 0.5 mg/kg, including serious adverse effects reported by the anaesthetists in 15% (bradycardia, cardiac arrhythmia). Tachycardia and laryngospasm were reported in 1 patient (3%). Parents reported difficulties breathing, pyrexia, and drowsiness in 14% (*182*). In the second trial (maximum dose 25 mg), restlessness was reported in 18/50 patients (36%), a higher incidence than with droperidol. Other adverse effects were similar to droperidol (*185*).

The Committee concluded that the evidence showed that promethazine is inferior to alternatives such as midazolam. The Committee recommended that promethazine be deleted from the EML.

Propofol (inclusion)

An application was prepared by Sharline Madera, William Shipman, Nicole Ramsey, and Professor Reidenberg, Weill Cornell Medical College, New York USA, for the addition of propofol to the Model List. Listing was requested as an individual medicine.

Expert reviews were prepared by Professor Abdol Majid Cheraghali and Professor David Ofori-Adjei. The Committee considered this application in conjunction with a review of the anaesthetic and muscle relaxant sections of the Model List and the application for the addition of midazolam for premedication and procedural sedation.

The Committee noted that propofol is widely used for the induction and maintenance of anaesthesia, and for sedation for short procedures. Evidence from two systematic reviews (*174*, *186*) and one narrative review (*187*) suggest that propofol, or propofol in combination with an opioid or isoflurane, has a quicker or similar rate of recovery and/or time to discharge than thiopental, sevoflurane, midazolam/nitrous oxide, thiopental/isoflurane/fentanyl/nitrous oxide, midazolam/opioid, diazepam, midazolam, hexobarbital/enflurane, thiopental/isoflurane, desflurane, or methohexital. The Committee noted that when compared to other IV induction anaesthetics, propofol was reported to have less or similar amounts of adverse effects (*174*, *187–189*). The Committee also considered evidence from two systematic reviews (*190*, *191*) that supported its safety and efficacy for paediatric procedural sedation and one RCT (*192*) for its use in paediatric ophthalmic procedures. The Committee noted that propofol is not recommended for obstetric procedures, caesarean sections, or deliveries.

The Committee noted that there is evidence to suggest that propofol is more cost effective than thiopental when use in ambulatory (day case) surgery due to shorter anaesthesia duration and faster recovery room stay (*193*, *194*).

The Committee acknowledged that there is high-quality evidence to support the safety and efficacy of propofol as an IV anaesthetic and that there are also potential cost benefits when used for day case surgery compared to thiopental. The Committee concluded that in settings where resources are sufficient to support a range of surgical services, including day case surgery, propofol is probably cost effective, although thiopental also needs to be available for certain indications. However in settings where surgical services and resources are limited, the IV anaesthetic of choice should be the one that is safe, effective, and can be used for the greatest number of indications, i.e. thiopental. The Committee noted increasing problems with availability of thiopental in some settings. The Committee recommended the addition of propofol to the Model List, and decided to list thiopental as an alternative, based on programmatic considerations (availability and cost).

Section 1.3: Preoperative medication and sedation for short-term procedures

Midazolam (inclusion)

An application was prepared by Dr Wildschut, Dr Nienke, and Dr de Wildt, Department of Pediatric Surgery and Intensive care, Erasmus MC Sophia

Children's Hospital, The Netherlands, for the inclusion of midazolam in Section 1.3 for both adults and children. Listing was requested as an individual medicine.

An expert review was prepared by Professor Hany Abdel-Aleem. Comments were received from Dr Bruce Reidenberg, Assistant Professor of Pharmacology and Pediatrics, Weill Cornell Medical College, New York.

The Committee considered evidence from a Cochrane systematic review (*195*) and 18 RCTs (*196–213*) in adults, a systematic review (*214*) and 22 RCTs (*213–236*) in children that supported the safety and efficacy of midazolam as premedication for a variety of surgical procedures. Only 1 of 19 RCTs in children, comparing midazolam to placebo, did not find a difference in depth of sedation or anxiety (*234*). One RCT in elderly patients (*198*) and five RCTs (*225, 227, 234–236*) in children suggested that midazolam prolonged discharge time, but that this did not lead to a prolonged hospital stay in the paediatric patients.

The use of midazolam has been associated with a decrease in postoperative nausea and vomiting after strabismus surgery (*237*) and tonsillectomy (*238*) in children. The Committee considered evidence from two systematic reviews (*188, 239*) in adults and seven RCTs in children to support the safety and efficacy of midazolam for sedation for short-term procedures (*240–246*). It was noted that in comparative studies midazolam had a similar efficacy to diazepam, but was associated with greater patient satisfaction and amnesic effect (*188*).

The Committee noted that a small percentage of children undergoing elective surgery have had paradoxical reactions following premedication with IV midazolam and that midazolam has been associated with longer recovery times in elderly patients and high-risk surgical patients, but that major adverse events are rare (*188, 247*).

The Committee noted that there were no cost–effectiveness studies comparing midazolam with diazepam.

Based on the large body of evidence to support the safety and efficacy of midazolam for premedication and procedural sedation, its wide availability and relatively low cost, the Committee recommended that midazolam should replace diazepam in Section 1.3 and be listed with a square box.

Section 4: Antidotes and other substances used in poisonings

Section 4.2: Specific

DL-methionine (deletion)

An application was prepared by Kristi Shiago, Isa Watson, and Professor Marcus Reidenberg, Weill Cornell Medical College, New York, USA for deletion of DL-methionine from the Model List.

Expert reviews were prepared by Professor Abdol Majid Cheraghali and Dr Kalle Hoppu.

The Committee considered evidence from one Cochrane Review (*248*) that reported that there were no head-to-head trials comparing N-acetylcysteine with DL-methionine but an indirect comparison based on pooled data from the individual studies suggested that acetylcysteine was slightly more effective. Both medicines have been used since the late 1970s and the safety profile is well established. The Committee noted that although the cost of methionine is lower than acetylcysteine, acetylcysteine has the advantage that it can be administered both orally and intravenously. The Committee was concerned that methionine may not be widely available as a single medicine in many countries, due to acetylcysteine having become the standard of care for paracetamol poisoning globally.

The Committee recommended the deletion of DL-methionine from the Model List due to its reported limited availability as a single medicine, the unknown real cost difference between DL-methionine and N-acetylcysteine, and the fact that N-acetylcysteine has become the standard of care globally for the treatment of paracetamol poisoning. DL-methionine has already been deleted from the EMLc.

Section 6: Anti-infective medicines

Section 6.2: Antibacterial medicines

Section 6.2.2: Other antibacterial medicines

Gatifloxacin (inclusion)

An application was prepared by Dr Piero Olliaro, Tropical Disease Research (TDR) Department, WHO, for the inclusion of gatifloxacin 200-mg and 400-mg solid oral dosage form for the treatment of enteric fever. Listing was requested as an individual medicine.

Expert reviews were completed by Professor Jennifer Welbeck and Professor Anita Zaidi. Comments were received from Dr Robert Peterson, Executive Director, Drug Safety and Effectiveness Network, Canadian Institutes of Health Research and Dr Bruce Reidenberg, Assistant Professor of Pharmacology and Pediatrics, Weill Cornell Medical College, New York.

The Committee noted that the estimated global burden of typhoid fever is 21 million cases annually with more than 210 000 deaths and paratyphoid fever is responsible for an additional 5 million cases (*249*); in endemic areas enteric fever is mainly a disease of young children and young adults and multidrug resistant and nalidixic acid resistant strains of *S. typhi* and *S. paratyphi* are increasing.

The Committee considered evidence from unpublished pharmacokinetic and pharmacodynamic studies by Dolocek et al. and three RCTs (*250–252*) to support the efficacy and safety of gatifloxacin for the treatment of enteric fever. The Committee noted that gatifloxacin has been associated with dysglycaemia, but the patients at risk appear to be elderly patients with age-related decreases in kidney function and non-insulin dependent diabetics on therapy. Patients with enteric fever are typically young children and young adults, who are unlikely to have non-insulin dependent diabetes and generally have good renal function. There is evidence from clinical trials to support the rarity of dysglycaemia in this population (*250–253*). The Committee noted that marketing approval for gatifloxacin has been withdrawn in a number of jurisdictions, including the United States, Canada, and India.

The Committee therefore recommended that gatifloxacin not be added to the Model List for the treatment of enteric fever because of safety concerns, the availability of alternatives, and the likelihood that supply will be limited in the future.

Isoniazid + pyridoxine + sulfamethoxazole + trimethoprim (new formulation)

The WHO Department of HIV has submitted a proposal for the inclusion of a new fixed-dose combination (FDC) containing isoniazid 300 mg, pyridoxine 25 mg, sulfamethoxazole 800 mg and trimethoprim 160 mg, for the prevention of TB and *Pneumocystis jiroveci* in adults living with HIV.

Expert reviews were provided by Professor Rohini Fernandopulle and Professor Abdol Majid Cheraghali.

The Committee noted that the proposal is generally consistent with WHO treatment guidelines for use of both isoniazid and sulfamethoxazole-pyrimethamine (co-trimoxazole). The application presents a summary of the clinical evidence as well as GRADE tables (grading of quality of scientific evidence) for the studies retrieved. All of the individual components are already included on the EML.

For co-trimoxazole, the review presents one RCT of 540 subjects that showed approximately a 30% reduction in mortality in patients with HIV who were treated compared to those who were not. The mean follow-up time for this study was 9.55 months. The study also found a reduction in cases of malaria, bacterial pneumonia, and isosporiasis in the treated group. Adverse events, based on four observational studies, were more frequent in the treated group.

For isoniazid, the review presents the result of eight RCTs (approximately 4000 subjects) in which patients were treated with 300 mg/day isoniazid or placebo. Patients treated with isoniazid had a statically significant reduction in the likelihood of confirmed TB. The relative risk for mortality was 0.95

(95% CI 0.85–1.06) favouring isoniazid; adverse reactions were slightly more frequent in the treated group. In three of these, pyridoxine 50 mg per day was co-administered with isoniazid.

There is no high-quality evidence concerning the impact of pyridoxine on isoniazid neurotoxicity other than the reversal of symptoms when the two are used in combination. The current practice is to use pyridoxine in patients with TB; the dose ranges from 25 mg per day to 50 mg per day.

The Committee noted that the product is not yet manufactured and no manufacturer has been identified. A report of a pharmaceutical feasibility study was provided that suggests the combination is technically feasible. There is no information about the potential cost of the combination product. Given the large amount of active pharmaceutical ingredients in the proposed FDC, formulation of an adequate product may result in a price that is higher than the existing loose combination.

The Committee decided that as the product does not yet exist, it cannot be added to the EML. The Committee decided to include it on a list of 'missing' essential medicines. Given that the new WHO Guidelines also recommend isoniazid and co-trimoxazole prophylaxis in children with HIV, a paediatric strength product also should be developed. The dose of isoniazid should be 10 mg/kg per day and the dose of co-trimoxazole needs to be determined.

Sulfamethoxazole + trimethoprim (new formulation)

The WHO Department of HIV has submitted a proposal for the inclusion of a new strength FDC containing sulfamethoxazole 800 mg and trimethoprim 160 mg, for the prevention of *P. jiroveci* in adults living with HIV. The proposal is generally consistent with WHO treatment guidelines for use of sulfamethoxazole-trimethoprim (co-trimoxazole). Several strengths of the FDC are already included on the EML.

Expert reviews were provided by Professor Abdol Majid Cheraghali and Professor Rohini Fernandopulle.

The application provides a summary of three clinical trials in adults infected with HIV, comparing treatment with sulfamethoxazole 800 mg and trimethoprim 160 mg with placebo. At 46 months, those receiving active treatment had a significantly lower risk of mortality compared with placebo (RR 0.65; 95% CI 0.56–0.76). The overall quality of evidence for the benefits of the intervention is assessed as high. Adverse events from treatment were not significantly different between the two groups. Costs for the FDC tablet range from US$ 0.0186 to US$ 0.0308 per day.

The Committee noted that the proposal is supported by the Director of the Stop TB Department, WHO.

The Committee recommended inclusion of the additional strength FDC on the EML.

Section 6.4: Antiviral medicines

Section 6.4.2: Antiretroviral medicines

The Committee took particular note of the WHO treatment guidelines for adults, which stated "There was no uncertainty among the panel concerning the need for third-line regimens. However, there was uncertainty about how making third-line regimens available would affect the provision of first-line and second-line ART. There was also uncertainty about what third-line drugs should be provided, as many studies are still in progress". The evidence submitted to the Expert Committee for all three antiretrovirals was not sufficient to allow for further definition of optimal third-line regimens, particularly considering a public health approach. The Committee therefore chose not to add any third-line antiretroviral agents to the List at this time, while being cognizant of the need to ensure that patients failing first- and second-line treatment have access to life-prolonging options. There is therefore an urgent need to identify a cost-effective public health approach to the choice of third-line antiretroviral treatments, for both adults and children.

Section 6.4.2.2: Non-nucleoside reverse transcriptase inhibitors

Etravirine (inclusion)

An application was submitted by Tibotec, an international pharmaceutical company, for the inclusion of etravirine (ETR) for the treatment of multidrug-resistant HIV-1 infection in adults.

Expert reviews of the application were prepared by Dr Gregory L Kearns, Mr Andy Gray, and Dr Lisa A Bero. Comments were received from the WHO Department of HIV and Dr Myriam Henkens, International Medical Coordinator, Médecins Sans Frontières.

The Committee considered the pooled 48-week data from 2 RCTs that supported the efficacy of etravirine in the treatment of multidrug-resistant HIV-1 in adults (*254*). The Committee noted that although the trials were multicentre and multinational, none of the trials took place in low-income settings and no children were included. The Committee also noted that although the incidence of adverse events and laboratory abnormalities were generally comparable to placebo at 48 weeks, development of a rash was significantly more common in the etravirine group. The Committee noted that there are many ongoing trials including trials in Africa, children and adolescents, lactating women, and drug interaction studies.

The Committee noted that economic evaluations undertaken in high-income countries have shown that the addition of etravirine to a regimen was associated with lower costs per person (with undetectable viral load) and lower hospital-related costs compared with placebo, but the results of these analyses are difficult to generalize to resource-poor settings (*255*).

On balance, due to the comparatively limited efficacy and long-term safety data for etravirine in adults and the lack of evidence in children and noting that there are many ongoing trials that might inform judgements about optimal combinations of antiretroviral agents for third-line therapy, the Committee recommended not to add etravirine to the Model List until more evidence in diverse populations and settings becomes available.

Section 6.4.2.3: Protease inhibitors

Darunavir (inclusion)

An application was submitted by Tibotec, an international pharmaceutical company, for the inclusion of darunavir for the treatment of multidrug-resistant HIV-1 infection in adults and children.

An expert review of the application was prepared by Dr Gregory L Kearns. Comments were received from the WHO Department of HIV and Dr Myriam Henkens, International Medical Coordinator, Médecins Sans Frontières.

The Committee considered evidence from four reports from two clinical trials (*256–259*) in adults and one observational study in children aged 6 to 17 years (*260*) that supported the efficacy of darunavir, in combination with low dose ritonavir, in the treatment of multidrug-resistant HIV-1. The adverse event profile of darunavir appeared similar to other frequently used protease inhibitors. The Committee noted that no data were available to support its use in pregnant women or children aged less than 6 years, and that the recommended dose of darunavir plus ritonavir for children in the 30 kg to <40 kg weight band would not be easy to administer with ritonavir products currently listed in the EMLc.

The Committee noted that darunavir has been registered in more than 60 countries and that economic evaluations in United States and European settings have indicated that darunavir/ritonavir-based highly active antiretroviral therapy (HAART) is cost effective compared with other standard of care protease inhibitor-based regimens in people living with HIV with evidence of protease inhibitor resistance (*261*).

Given the relatively limited evidence of efficacy, safety, and cost–effectiveness in both adults and children in a diversity of settings, that the optimal use of darunavir is still being defined, and uncertainty regarding the best combinations of medicines for third-line regimens, the Committee recommended that darunavir should not be added to the Complementary List. Further development of darunavir is clearly required, including fixed-dose combination products of darunavir/ritonavir especially for children.

Section 6.4.2.4: Integrase inhibitors (new section heading)

Raltegravir (inclusion)

An application was submitted by Amitabh Suther (consultant), on behalf of the WHO Department of HIV, for the treatment of multidrug-resistant HIV-1 infection in adults.

An expert review of the application was prepared by Dr Lisa A Bero. Comments were received from the WHO Department of HIV and Dr Myriam Henkens, International Medical Coordinator, Médecins Sans Frontières.

The Committee considered evidence from four reports of two clinical trials in adults (*262–265*) that supported the efficacy of raltegravir in the treatment of multidrug-resistant HIV-1 in patients aged 16 years and older. The adverse event profile of raltegravir was similar to placebo. The Committee noted that no data were available to support its use in pregnant women or children and that there were no cost–effectiveness data available for raltegravir.

Given the relatively limited evidence of efficacy, safety and cost–effectiveness in both adults and children in a diversity of settings and that the optimal use of raltegravir is still being defined as well as the best combinations of medicines for third-line regimens, the Committee recommended that raltegravir should not be added to the Complementary List. As with darunavir, further development of the product is clearly required, especially with respect to its possible use in children aged less than 16 years.

Section 6.5: Antiprotozoal medicines

Section 6.5.2: Antileishmaniasis medicines

Miltefosine (inclusion) – Adults and children

An application was submitted by Paladin Labs Barbados, the manufacturer of miltefosine, for its inclusion on the WHO Model List of Essential Medicines for the treatment of cutaneous and visceral leishmaniasis in adults and children. A previous application was considered in 2005 but at that time, the Committee did not recommend its inclusion due to lack of information about the pharmacokinetic profile in humans; a lack of efficacy and safety data for the treatment of cutaneous leishmaniasis; a lack of dosing information and safety data for its use in visceral leishmaniasis; and the need for comparative cost–effectiveness data, including a comparison with liposomal amphotericin B.

Expert reviews were provided by Dr Kalle Hoppu and Professor Anita Zaidi. The Committee noted the numerous comments from individuals and organizations supporting the application.

The application does not provide a search strategy or reference existing systematic reviews. Data were presented in relation to visceral leishmaniasis (6 studies, 2 of which were RCTs), cutaneous leishmaniasis (4 studies, including

3 RCTs) and mucosal leishmaniasis (1 observational study). In visceral leishmaniasis, miltefosine was superior to amphotericin B, and similar to antimony but less toxic; in the studies in cutaneous leishmaniasis, miltefosine was superior to placebo and similar or superior to antimonials, again with less toxicity. The Committee noted that there were no comparative trials of miltefosine with either liposomal amphotericin B or paromomycin.

For combination treatment, the evidence is based on one trial very recently published in the *Lancet* (*266*). This was a randomized four-arm comparison of amphotericin B (n=157), miltefosine + liposomal amphotericin B (n=160), paromomycin + liposomal amphotericin B (n=155), or miltefosine + paromomycin (n=158). The trial was designed as a non-inferiority comparison and on the basis of the per-protocol analysis there was no difference between the treatment options. On the basis of the intention to treat population, all combinations are probably superior to conventional amphotericin alone.

The Committee noted that studies in animals have shown reproductive toxicity so that miltefosine is currently contraindicated for use in pregnant women. The European Medicines Agency (EMA) has assessed the risk of teratogenic effects as requiring women of childbearing potential to use effective contraception during and up to three months after treatment. Paladin's pharmacovigilance group has received no reports of any birth defects since the first regulatory approval of miltefosine. From November 2004 until March 2009, 62 659 treatment courses have been supplied either for clinical trials, government treatment programmes, or individual use.

Evidence showing the comparative cost–effectiveness of current leishmaniasis treatment strategies was comprehensively summarized in the application. The data presented suggest that treatment with miltefosine is the least expensive, with the exception of paromomycin.

The Committee was informed that the Department of Control of Neglected Tropical Diseases held a WHO Expert Committee Meeting on Leishmaniasis in 2010 (published as *WHO Technical Report Series*, No. 949). The report of the meeting includes many recommendations on treatment, including recommendations on the use of miltefosine. It also recommends the use of combination treatment for visceral leishmaniasis. This report is the basis of the recommendation from the Department for inclusion of miltefosine in the WHO Model List. The Department has also recommended that a note be included in the List that for visceral leishmaniasis caused by *L. donovani*, miltefosine, paromomycin, and antimonials should only be used in combination therapy. The report of the Expert Committee does not provide full details of the basis for the recommendation as it does not contain references.

Based on evidence of efficacy and safety in the treatment of visceral leishmaniasis in both adults and children, and evidence of efficacy and safety in the treatment of adults in cutaneous and mucosal leishmaniasis, the Committee decided to add miltefosine to the WHO Model List for both adults and children. Due to the teratogenic risks of miltefosine treatment a note should be added to the listing indicating that it should not be used in women of childbearing age unless contraception can be guaranteed for the duration of treatment and three months afterwards. The Committee did not recommend a note concerning combination treatment until there is more evidence of the potential advantages over single component treatment. The Committee was informed about agreements on a pricing structure and preferential pricing for developing countries. Compliance with this agreement needs to be monitored.

Section 6.5.3: Antimalarial medicines

Artesunate + amodiaquine fixed-dose combination (inclusion) – Adults and children

Artesunate and amodiaquine (AS+AQ) have been recommended by WHO as one of the preferred artemisinin combination treatments for malaria since the WHO treatment guidelines published in 2006. Sanofi-Aventis has submitted an updated application to list the fixed-dose combination product containing ASAQ in three different strengths: 25 mg+67.5 mg, 50 mg+135 mg, and 100 mg+270 mg. The application was first considered by the Subcommittee in 2007, and subsequently by the Expert Committee in October 2007. The application was rejected because of uncertainty about the dose of amodiaquine in the FDC compared to the usually recommended dose, the relatively premature nature of the presentation of one of the key clinical trials and the uncertainty about the availability of a quality-assured product.

The current application, based on the regulatory dossier for the Sanofi-Aventis product, was submitted in June 2009, and updated again in October 2010, to reflect changes in the new WHO treatment guidelines (2010 edition) and updated information about licensing. The Sanofi-Aventis product was approved as prequalified by WHO at the end of 2008. It is licensed in several African countries and in India.

Expert reviews were provided by Professor Jennifer Welbeck and Mr Andy Gray.

As in 2007, there are two studies in the application that use the proposed FDC: the Burkina Faso study (*267*), which is a comparison of the FDC with a loose combination in a different dose, and the ATAQ EASY study (*268*), comparing the FDC with artemether + lumefantrine (AL). A complete overview of comparative effectiveness studies is provided in the Cochrane Review by Sinclair et al. (*269*) and the (unpublished) 2011 update of this review has been completed and provided to the Committee. It includes:

- 2 trials of AS+AQ versus DHA-PPQ (day 28 data are available from 2 trials, day 42 from 1 trial);
- 1 trial of AS+AQ versus AS+MQ (day 28 data only);

- 12 trials of AS+AQ 6 doses of artemether + lumefantrine (polymerase chain reaction (PCR)-adjusted day 28 data are available from 11 trials, day 42 from 1 trial; 3 further trials excluded due to baseline differences);
- 7 trials of AS+AQ versus AS+SP (day 28 data only); and
- 9 trials of AS+AQ versus AQ+SP (PCR-adjusted day 28 data available from 7 trials).

When assessing AS+AQ compared to other artemisinin combination therapies, the updated results from the Cochrane Review for the comparisons of the outcome day 28 PCR treatment failure are:

- AS+AQ versus DHA-PPQ: 2 studies, 329 subjects, pooled RR 2.36 (95% CI 0.74–7.54), favours DHA-PPQ;
- AS+AQ versus AL: 11 studies, 2791 participants: RR 0.65 (95% CI 0.40–1.04), favours AS+AQ; and
- AS+AQ versus AS+MQ: 1 study, 482 subjects, 0 events so comparative relative risk not estimable.

In terms of comparative safety, the information in the application has been updated by a safety review, prepared by a member of the Advisory Committee on the Safety of Medicines, that identifies adverse drug reactions suggestive of extra-pyramidal reactions in adults consistent with previous similar reports noted with amodiaquine monotherapy. No other new information concerning safety has been identified.

The Committee noted that the current WHO treatment guidelines recommend a target dose of 4 mg/kg per day of artesunate (therapeutic range 2–10 mg/kg per day) and 10 mg/kg per day (range 7.5–15 mg/kg per day). A proportion of potential 'weight bands' receive less than the target dose of 4 mg/kg per day artesunate but more than the minimum of 2 mg/kg per day. Doubling the dose usually results in excess amodiaquine with the resultant risk of increased toxicity. The trials provided show that the FDC appears to have similar efficacy compared with the loose combination at a slightly different dose. The Committee was assured by the relevant WHO department that the doses delivered were considered appropriate to deliver at least 2 mg/kg per day of artesunate. The FDC composition had been included in WHO treatment guidelines and there were WHO prequalified products available for the FDCs proposed.

The Committee decided to include the proposed FDCs on the EML and EMLc, but with a note specifying that appropriate doses may also be achievable using combinations of the monocomponent products, including as co-blistered presentations. The mono-component amodiaquine cannot be deleted as a separate listing in the EML, but the note needs to be consistent with existing guidelines for the treatment of *Plasmodium vivax*, *P. ovale* and *P. malariae* malaria.

Dihydroartemisinin + piperaquine (inclusion) – Adults and children

Dihydroartemisinin and piperaquine (DHA+PPQ) have been recommended by WHO as one of the preferred artemisinin combination treatments for malaria in the WHO treatment guidelines published in 2010. The Committee considered an application from Sigma-Tau for a FDC product in two strengths: 40 mg DHA + 320 mg PPQ and 20 mg DHA + 160 mg PPQ. Target doses for the components, as stated in the 2010 WHO treatment guidelines are: 4 mg/kg per day DHA (range 2–10 mg/kg per day) and 18 mg/kg per day PPQ (range 16–26 mg/kg per day).

Reviews of the application were prepared by Dr Lisa A Bero and Professor Jennifer Welbeck.

The application is a summary of the regulatory dossier for the Sigma-Tau product and does not include a search for other literature. It refers to 6 PK studies (4 in healthy volunteers) and 2 open-label randomized Phase III studies that compared DHA+PPQ to artesunate mefloquine in Asia and to artemether+AL in Africa. Both studies were designed as non-inferiority studies, with the primary outcome being day 63 PCR-corrected cure rates.

The Asian study enrolled 1150 subjects, aged between six months and 62 years (median age 25 years). The African study enrolled 1553 patients, aged between 6 and 59 months (median age 2.42 years). Results from these studies showed that DHA+PPQ was non-inferior to both other treatments.

The Committee considered the information from an update of the Cochrane Review on artemisinin combination therapies. It includes:

- 10 trials of DHA+PPQ versus AS+MQ (day 28 data are available from 7 trials, day 63 from 5 trials);
- 9 trials of DHA+PPQ versus 6 doses of artemether + lumefantrine (day 28 data are available from 7 trials, day 42 from 7 trials, day 63 from 1 trial);
- 2 trials of DHA+PPQ versus AS+AQ (day 28 data are available from 2 trials, day 42 from 1 trial);
- 1 trial of DHA+PPQ versus AS+sulfadoxine-pyrimethamine (day 28 and day 42 data available); and
- 2 trials of DHA+PPQ versus AQ+SP (day 28 data available from 2, day 42 from 1).

However, the studies in the application do not appear to have been included in the Cochrane Review.

On the basis of the studies presented, the FDC proposed for the EML appears to be at least non-inferior to other artemisinin combination therapies. However, the overall data set of studies needs to be fully evaluated to be certain about what differences exist, if any, between DHA-PPQ and other artemisinin combination therapies. In terms of comparative safety, the information in the application is based on the Sigma-Tau database of 8 clinical trials and data from an additional 4590 subjects and 26 additional studies identified in the literature. Adverse events thought to be related to treatment include nausea, asthenia, dizziness, influenza, and anorexia. QT prolongation has been investigated at the request of the EMA, resulting in the recommendation to take the product before food.

The current WHO treatment guidelines recommend a target dose of 4 mg/kg per day of DHA (therapeutic range 2–10 mg/kg per day) and 18 mg/mg per day of PPQ (range 16–26 mg/kg per day). The Committee considered the actual dose that would be delivered per kg based on the recommended dosing regimens for the different strength FDCs and noted with concern that none of the weight bands receive the target dose of DHA; all receive less than 4 mg/kg per day.

No actual cost data are provided. The application states that DHA-PPQ will be comparable in price to other artemisinin combination therapies.

The Committee noted that this product is available, but has not yet been approved by any stringent authority and that a decision by the EMA has been deferred until April 2011. It was not clear whether this decision was based on concerns about efficacy, safety, or quality. The overall assessment of comparative effectiveness and safety is hampered by what appear to be several large unpublished trials not yet in the public domain. The safety data presented do not allow a full assessment of comparative safety. The FDC when given according to the recommended regimen does not deliver target doses of the components, as noted in the WHO treatment guidelines.

The Committee therefore recommended that the application should be deferred, pending a comprehensive summary of all existing clinical trials, as well as an assessment of the evidence for the efficacy of the target doses of the components compared to dose delivered. The Committee requested that this review be carried out urgently. An extra session of the Committee could be convened before the next scheduled meeting to make a recommendation on this FDC.

Pyronaridine + artesunate fixed-dose combination (inclusion) – Adults and children

Shin Poon Pharmaceutical Co. Ltd has submitted an application for a new fixed-dose combination for malaria, containing pyronaridine and artesunate (Py-AS). The product has been developed in partnership with Medicines for Malaria Venture, as a three-day course of treatment for both *falciparum* and *vivax* malaria infections. The product is not yet on the market and is under review by the EMA. It is not yet recommended in the WHO treatment guideline for malaria.

Expert reviews were prepared by Dr Lisa A Bero and Professor Rohini Fernandopulle.

The Committee noted that the application is based on the regulatory dossier for the product developed by Shin Poon. The clinical evidence consists of brief summaries of the unpublished Phase II and Phase III studies: two dose-finding studies – 1 each in adults and children – and 4 comparative studies: Py-AS versus AS-MQ, 2 with Py-AS versus AL, and Py-AS versus chloroquine. One of the AL comparative studies has been published as Tshefu et al. 2010 (*270*); and the chloroquine study has also been published as Poravuth Y et al. (*271*). The other studies have not yet been published.

Based on the main trial so far, Tshefu et al. (*270*), Py-AS appears to be non-inferior in terms of efficacy in falciparum malaria. However, given the relatively limited information about the unpublished trials in the application, it is clear that the additional results need to be provided before a full assessment can be made. The Cochrane Review contains additional single component trials, but no other trials of the FDC.

The application provides a brief assessment of comparative safety. Of note is the effect on liver enzymes, as documented in the published trial reports. In Tshefu et al. (*270*), 8 patients receiving Py-AS were recorded as having grade 3 or grade 4 toxicity for liver enzymes rises, compared to 1 in the AL group; in Poravuth et al., 3 in the Py-AS group had liver enzyme changes compared with 0 in the chloroquine group. The application states that the findings and rapid resolution are consistent with direct, low-level toxicity and do not indicate a risk of progressive liver injury.

The Committee considered this application to be premature. The product is not yet available, there are additional clinical data that will become available and there is a safety issue that needs to be resolved. The Committee decided to reject the application at this time, and to invite re-submission once the outstanding issues have been resolved.

Section 8: Antineoplastic agents, immunosuppressives, and medicines used in palliative care

Section 8.2: Cytotoxic medicines

Paclitaxel (inclusion)

Docetaxel (inclusion)

An application was prepared by the NHS Centre for the Evaluation of Effectiveness of Health Care, Emilia Romagna Regional Health System, Modena,

Italy, at the request of the Secretariat for the Expert Committee for the Selection and Use of Essential Medicines for the inclusion of a taxane on the Model List.

Expert reviews of the application were prepared by Dr Lisa A Bero and Professor Noël Cranswick.

The Committee noted that the application provided a comprehensive review of the available evidence. The application cited 1 systematic review (*272*) supporting the use of taxanes (paclitaxel or docetaxel) in the treatment of metastatic breast cancer and 2 systematic reviews (*273*, *274*) supporting their use in the treatment of early breast cancer in adjuvant settings. The use of a taxane-containing regimen improved disease free survival and overall survival compared to a non-taxane containing regimen in the treatment of both early and advanced breast cancer. When the studies for docetaxel and paclitaxel were analysed separately, they showed similar results for overall survival and disease free survival in breast cancer. However, paclitaxel is also used in the treatment of ovarian cancer (*275*).

The toxicity profiles of paclitaxel and docetaxel were similar; both can cause bone marrow suppression and hypersensitivity reactions. The Committee highlighted that they should only be administered in a facility equipped to manage possible complications.

The Committee considered a review of cost–effectiveness data prepared by the Secretariat. This evidence suggested that docetaxel may be more cost effective than paclitaxel in the treatment of advanced or metastatic breast cancer, an important consideration for low- and middle-income countries, where breast cancer is often diagnosed at a more advanced stage.

Overall, the Committee acknowledged that the evidence provided in the application supports the public health need and comparable effectiveness and safety of taxanes for the treatment of early and advanced breast cancer. Although not specifically addressed in the application, there is good evidence of the efficacy of paclitaxel in the treatment of ovarian cancer. Views expressed by the WHO Department of Chronic Diseases, Prevention and Management, which did not support inclusion, on the basis of concerns about diversion of attention and resources from screening efforts, were noted.

After taking into consideration the available data, the Committee recommended the inclusion of both docetaxel and paclitaxel on the Complementary List.

Section 10: Medicines affecting the blood

Section 10.2: Medicines affecting coagulation

Tranexamic acid (inclusion)

In 2009, the Committee considered an application for the addition of tranexamic acid to the EML, but rejected it because the major indication proposed was for use to reduce blood loss in cardiac surgery. This indication was considered to be of uncertain public health relevance.

In 2010, the report of a large RCT (*276*) comparing tranexamic acid to placebo in the treatment of adult patients with trauma and at significant risk of ongoing haemorrhage was published. One of the authors of the trial, Professor Ian Roberts, has resubmitted the application based on the results of the study. The revised application now targets the use of tranexamic acid for trauma patients. As noted in the application, road traffic accidents are the ninth leading cause of death globally. It is proposed that listing tranexamic acid will contribute to a reduction in this cause of death, as well as reduce the need for blood transfusion for the management of trauma patients.

Expert reviews have been prepared by Mr Andy Gray and Professor Rohini Fernandopulle. Many letters of support for the inclusion of tranexamic acid have been submitted, including many from trial contributors. The WHO Department of Violence and Injury Prevention supported the inclusion of tranexamic acid.

The Committee noted that intravenous tranexamic acid is licensed in a number of countries for short-term use as prophylaxis and treatment in surgery; for the treatment of haemorrhagic complications associated with thrombolytic therapy; disseminated intravascular coagulation; and hereditary angioneurotic oedema, but it has not yet been approved for use in trauma.

As noted above, the main additional evidence in this application is the CRASH-2 trial. This large (n=20211) double blind multi centre RCT (40 countries) is described in detail in the application. The results for the primary outcome, in-hospital mortality within four weeks of injury were that patients treated with tranexamic acid had a reduced risk of death (all-cause mortality) (RR 0.91; 95% CI 0.85–0.97) as well as reduced risk of death due to bleeding (RR 0.85; 95% CI 0.76–0.96). Vascular occlusive events were not different between the two groups. There was no difference in transfusion requirements between the two groups, either in terms of number of patients receiving transfusions or the amount of blood products actually used.

The Committee considered that the quality of the trial is high.

The Committee noted that it is not clear from the trial what degree of specialist monitoring is required for safe use of tranexamic acid. European trauma guidelines recommend monitoring of fibrinolysis in all trauma patients to guide treatment. The Committee noted that the use of tranexamic acid should not replace appropriate provision of blood transfusions. There are no data to establish efficacy and safety in children.

The Committee evaluated the information provided about comparative cost and cost–effectiveness. The application provides a sample of prices for tranexamic acid, ranging from US$ 2.57 per gram to US$ 22.83 per gram. The application presents the summary of a (yet unpublished) cost–effectiveness analysis based on the trial, adjusted for estimated survival gains in different settings and the age distribution of trauma patients in each setting. The assumptions are not provided in sufficient detail to independently verify them. Simple estimates of incremental cost per death averted based on the observed risk difference and 95% CI in the trial and drug costs alone, and with low and high costs are shown in Table 4.

Table 4
Estimates of incremental cost per death averted for tranexamic acid

	Low	Numbers needed to treat	High
Cost/g	US$ 41	US$ 68	US$ 206
US$ 2.57	210.74	349.52	1058.84
US$ 22.83	1872.06	3104.88	9405.96

Overall, the Committee noted that use of tranexamic acid is likely to be cost effective in settings where the baseline mortality from trauma is at least that in the trial (15%) and where there are facilities for administration of tranexamic acid early following injury, especially if the product can be purchased at prices lower than US$ 10/g. If the baseline risk of mortality is lower, with a resultant NNT between 100 and 200, it is important that the price paid for the product is kept as low as possible to ensure cost–effectiveness and affordability.

The Committee therefore recommended addition to the Core List. The Committee recommended that an evidence summary be provided on the web site including the cost–effectiveness data to allow countries to make procurement decisions considering best available prices for products of adequate quality.

Section 12: Cardiovascular medicines

Bisoprolol (inclusion) – square box

An application was prepared by Pharmacy Students: Sandeep Kishore, Maryam Shafaee, Mathew Price, and Rajesh Vedanthan, and Marcus Reidenberg, Professor of Pharmacology, Medicine and Public Health, New York, for the addition of bisoprolol with a square box to the Model List, replacing atenolol as the representative medicine of the class in Sections 12.1 to 12.3, and the inclusion of beta-blockers as a therapeutic class in Section 14.4 (Medicines used in heart failure). Listing is requested as a representative of its therapeutic class.

Expert reviews were prepared by Dr Lenita Wannmacher and Professor Rohini Fernandopulle. Comments were received from Dr Shanti Mendis, Coordinator, Chronic Diseases Prevention and Management, WHO, and Dr Prabhakaran, Executive Director, Centre for Chronic Disease Control, New Dehli, India.

The Committee noted that heart failure is an important global health issue and its prevalence is increasing worldwide due to both communicable and noncommunicable causes. Recent guidelines from the National Institute of Clinical Excellence (NICE), United Kingdom, and Heart Failure Society of America (HSFA) recommend beta-blockers for the treatment of heart failure and specifically cite metoprolol, bisoprolol, and carvedilol (*277*, *278*).

The Committee considered evidence from 3 RCTs (*279–281*) to support the efficacy and safety of the beta-blockers bisoprolol, metoprolol, and carvedilol in the treatment of heart failure, as well as 3 meta-analyses that found a reduction of 29% to 34% in the composite end-point of mortality or hospital admission with beta-blocker therapy in patients with heart failure (*282–284*). Mortality benefits have been shown in diverse patient groups, including the elderly (*285*), patients with diabetes (*281*) and without (*286*), patients with an ejection fraction above or below 25% (*287*) and patients not receiving rennin-angiotensin inhibitors (*288*); additionally bisoprolol can be used in patients with chronic obstructive pulmonary disease (*289*). The Committee noted that there is no high-quality evidence to support the use of atenolol for the treatment of heart failure.

The Committee noted that there is evidence from clinical trials to support the efficacy and safety of bisoprolol for the treatment of angina (*290*, *291*) arrhythmias (*279*, *292–294*), and hypertension (*295–297*). The Committee also took into consideration a meta-analysis (*298*) (5 studies, n=17671, follow-up 4.6 years) that suggested older hypertensive patients treated with atenolol have a significantly higher mortality when compared to patients treated with other classes of cardiovascular medicines. Cardiovascular mortality was also higher in the atenolol treated group than with other antihypertensive treatment, and strokes were more frequent with atenolol treatment.

The Committee noted that on a cost per dose basis bisoprolol was cheaper than metoprolol and carvedilol.

The Committee concluded that there was sufficient evidence of efficacy and safety compared to atenolol to support the request for bisoprolol to become the representative beta-blocker in sections 12.1 to 12.3 and also recommended, based on evidence of efficacy, safety, and cost–effectiveness, that bisoprolol should be added to the Model List for the treatment of heart failure. Due to the similarities between bisoprolol and metoprolol in terms of efficacy, the Committee decided to add bisoprolol with a square box for this indication. It was noted that country programmes could choose between bisoprolol, metoprolol, or carvedilol, but that there were increasingly reasons not to select atenolol as the sole beta-blocker provided.

Section 13: Dermatological medicines (topical)

Dermatological medicines (review) – Adults and children

A review of the dermatological medicines currently listed on the WHO Model List of Essential Medicines was prepared by the International League of Dermatology Societies (ILDS) in response to recommendations made by the Subcommittee (October 2008).

The review made the following recommendations:

- addition of terbinafine cream or ointment;
- deletion of benzoic acid + salicylic acid;
- addition of tetracycline 3% ointment or mupirocin or fucidin cream;
- deletion of neomycin + bacitracin;
- deletion of methylrosanilinium chloride (gentian violet);
- consider addition of an intermediate strength steroid;
- deletion of aluminium diacetate;
- deletion of dithranol;
- addition of 5% urea;
- addition of topical sulfur containing preparations 2–5%; and
- addition of itraconazole for the treatment of deep fungal infections, including chromoblastomycosis, histoplasmosis, paracoccidioidomycosis, and infections due to *Penicillium mameffei* as an alternative to amphotericin B (use restricted to severe, advanced disease).

Expert reviews were prepared by Professor Abdol Majid Cheraghali and Dr Gregory L Kearns.

The Committee noted that although terbinafine ointment is reported to be more effective than 1% azoles for the treatment of tinea pedis, the evidence provided in the review was not sufficient to support this claim. It is relatively expensive, but is increasingly available from generic sources. On balance, the Committee decided to recommend the inclusion of terbinafine and the deletion of Whitfield ointment (benzoic acid and salicylic acid ointment).

Topical tetracycline is widely available and used for the management of superficial skin infections, but there is limited evidence to support its efficacy and safety in children and drug resistance is a concern, especially in communities where tetracycline eye ointment has been widely used. The Committee noted that there is evidence from a Cochrane systematic review (*299*) to support the safety and efficacy of mupirocin and fucidin for topical treatment of superficial bacterial infections. Although the availability of mupirocin has in the past been limited, acquisition costs are falling as generic forms enter the market. The Cochrane Review also highlighted the risk of allergic reactions to preparations containing neomycin. No information about the use of topical antibacterials in neonates was identified. The Committee decided to delete neomycin and bacitracin, and replace this with mupirocin.

The Committee noted that there is evidence that gentian violet may act as a carcinogen (*300, 301*). Although noting that this agent is widely used as an antifungal and antiseptic, the Committee decide to delete gentian violet from the List.

The review did not identify any data to support the use of aluminium diacetate as an astringent and did not identify any areas where it is widely used. This item was therefore deleted from the List.

The Committee noted that dithranol was deleted from the WHO Model List for Children in 2009 and that there are safety concerns with its use. The Committee did not, however, feel that there were sufficient data at hand to allow for a decision on replacement for dithranol for adults, and therefore called for a review of this section before the next meeting.

There are few published data for the use of sulfur containing preparations for human scabies. Two small studies (n≤10) support the safety of topical sulfur containing preparations in children aged less than 1 year (*302, 303*).

Itraconazole has been studied in RCTs, but a formal review of these has not been undertaken. The Committee therefore did not make any changes to the List in respect of antifungals for deep infections.

The Committee noted that the review highlights the safety concerns with the use of lindane in children; it has been associated with convulsions in young children and with aplastic anaemia. Lindane was deleted from the WHO Model List in 1992 on the grounds of toxicity and the presence of safer alternatives on the List. The Committee therefore decided to retain permethrin and not to add lindane.

The Committee accepted the recommendation to change the strength of urea listed to 5–10%, instead of 10% only.

Lastly, the Committee did not make any changes to the corticosteroid cream listed.

Section 17: Gastrointestinal medicines

Section: 17.1: Antacids and other anti-ulcer medicines

Aluminium hydroxide (deletion)

Magnesium hydroxide (deletion)

An application was prepared by Professor Abdol Majid Cheraghali for the deletion of aluminium hydroxide and magnesium hydroxide from the Model List.

Expert reviews were prepared by Dr Kalle Hoppu and Dr Lenita Wannmacher. Comments were received from Dr Shanti Mendis, Coordinator, Chronic Diseases Prevention and Management, Médecins Sans Frontières, and Dr S Manikandan, Assistant Professor of Pharmacology, Mahatma Gandhi Medical College and Research Institute, Pondicherry, India.

The Committee considered evidence from one Cochrane systematic review that indicated antacids are no better than placebo for the treatment of dyspepsia (*304*).

The Committee recommended the deletion of antacids from the Model List, for both adults and children, due to evidence of no benefit compared to placebo and the presence of safe and effective alternative medicines for the treatment of gastro-oesophageal reflux disease and non-ulcer dyspepsia in adults, including pregnant women, on the Model List. The Committee recommended that a review be commissioned to consider the possible deletion of rantidine from the List, and the retention of omeprazole instead. This review should also consider the need for a parenteral dosage form in this regard.

Review of treatment of Helicobacter pylori *in adults and children*

In 2009, omeprazole was added to the EML, and the Expert Committee requested a review of medicines for the treatment of *Helicobacter pylori*. Currently, the EML includes omeprazole with a square box, amoxicillin, erythromycin, and metronidazole, used in combination to eradicate *H. Pylori*. Azithromycin, an alternative antibiotic in some regimens, is listed for infections by *Chlamydia trachomatis* only. Clarithromycin and tinidazole are not listed. Tetracyclines are listed as eye ointment only. Fluoroquinolones are listed (ciprofloxacin, ofloxacin, levofloxacin).

An expert review was prepared by Dr Lenita Wannmacher and reviewed by Dr Lisa A Bero and Professor Anita Zaidi. Dr Shanti Mendis, Coordinator from the WHO Chronic Diseases Prevention and Management Department, supported the inclusion of clarithromycin to be used in standard triple therapy.

H. pylori infection is the main cause of peptic ulcer. Infection is acquired in infancy and remains life-long unless treated. Approximately half of the world's population is infected by *H. pylori*, but most have no symptoms or significant complications.

The review provided was comprehensive. The Committee noted that there were relatively few data in children.

The Committee reviewed the indications where *H. pylori* eradication has shown benefits. There is high-quality evidence of benefit of eradication of *H. pylori* in treatment of peptic ulcer as well as in prevention of ulcer recurrence (*305*); eradication produced long-term cure in more than 80% of patients with duodenal ulcers not associated with NSAIM use. There is no evidence of benefit in patients on long-term NSAIM (*306*). There is also evidence that *H. pylori* eradication can reduce recurrent bleeding in patients with bleeding ulcers (*307*).

However, the evidence of benefit is less clear in patients with non-ulcer dyspepsia, and gastro-oesophageal reflux (*308*). Despite strong epidemiological links between *H. pylori* infection and gastric cancer, there was conflicting evidence on the benefit of *H. pylori* eradication on cancer prevention.

The Committee considered the evidence supporting combination regimens for *H. pylori* eradication. International guidelines (North America and European Union) recommend a triple combination of a proton pump inhibitor (PPI) or ranitidine bismuth citrate, and two of three antibiotics (amoxicillin, clarithromycin, or metronidazole) for adults or children. Guidelines do differ in treatment duration: 10–14 days in North America and 7 days in the European Union (*309, 310*).

For duration of treatment, a comparison of 7 days, 10 days, or 14 days showed no benefit of extending treatment beyond 7 days (*311*).

The Committee then assessed different components of the treatment regimens to determine what should be added to the EML.

Based on several meta-analyses, the Committee concluded that PPIs are similarly effective for *H. pylori* eradication when combined with a variety of different antibiotics. The Committee considered that there was no evidence of differences in efficacy among PPIs (esomeprazole, omeprazole, pantoprazole), but differences in safety profiles, omeprazole and pantoprazole being better tolerated than esomeprazole or rabeprazole. The Committee acknowledged that PPIs have different costs, not supported by differences in effectiveness, and may represent significant costs in health care budgets. The Committee therefore confirmed that omeprazole with a square box be maintained in the EML.

The Committee noted that amoxicillin given twice daily is as effective as four times daily (2 g/day) for *H. pylori* eradication (*312*). In children a dose of 50 mg/kg per day was found effective. In case of penicillin allergy, substitution with clarithromycin or a quinolone is possible.

Among macrolides, clarithromycin and azithromycin, but not erythromycin, have been studied in *H. pylori* infections. The Committee noted that *H. pylori* resistance to clarithromycin has increased, which may be explaining decreased cure rates (<80%) after first-line therapy. A study performed in Tunisia showed resistance levels of 14.6% and 56.8% in adults, and 18.8% and 25% in children for clarithromycin and metronidazole, respectively (*313*). The choice of first-line treatment should therefore be based on local resistance patterns. Clarithromycin doses of 500 mg twice daily (or modified release 1 g/day) have been used successfully for *H. pylori* eradication, but a comparison of doses of 400 mg and 800 mg per day produced similar cure rates. In children a dose of 15 mg/kg has been found effective.

Azithromycin-based regimens may have advantages in terms of adverse events but there is some uncertainty concerning efficacy. The Committee noted the high level of *H. pylori* resistance to tetracycline in studies (up to 38% in a study in Iran in 2009) which may reduce its potential benefit.

Costs of treatment were evaluated. In developed countries, a comparison of different triple therapies to H_2 antagonists maintenance was conducted. Although a bismuth-based triple therapy for 14 days was cheaper than a PPI-based triple therapy for 7 days, both were cheaper and more effective (US$ 223–410, with recurrence prevention of 70–86%) than H_2 antagonists maintenance (US$ 425, 72% recurrence prevention) (*314*). Other data show that two regimens were the most cost effective (compared to four other combinations), a triple combination of omeprazole, clarithromycin, and amoxicillin, and a quadruple one of ranitidine, metronidazole, amoxicillin, and bismuth, producing eradication rates and costs of 90% at €195.8, and 90% at €158.7, respectively (*315*). From International Buyer Prices, a 7-day clarithromycin treatment (1 g/day) would cost between approximately US$ 5.52 and US$ 6 and omeprazole (20 mg/day) about US$ 0.92 (price in Costa Rica).

The Committee reviewed the evidence relating to bismuth salts. The inclusion of bismuth in a triple combination (with tetracycline and PPI) resulted in higher cure rates than a triple combination (clarithromycin with amoxicillin and PPI) but more severe adverse effects were reported in the bismuth group (*316*). The Committee noted that the addition of bismuth could overcome clarithromycin resistance in quadruple combinations. However, the Committee also considered that the availability of bismuth salts was limited in many countries, where regulatory action has resulted in its withdrawal for safety reasons.

In summary, the Committee concluded that clarithromycin should be added to the EML, specifically for use in *H. pylori* eradication regimens, that metronidazole should be maintained on the List for this purpose in addition to the existing indications, but that there was no reason to include bismuth salts or azithromycin at this time. There was insufficient evidence of clinical benefit to justify inclusion on the EMLc at this time. Choice of treatment regimen should be based on national guidelines, with due consideration of local resistance patterns, availability, and cost.

Section 17.5: Medicines used in diarrhoea

Section 17.5.3: Antidiarrhoeal (symptomatic) medicines in adults

Codeine (deletion)

Loperamide (inclusion)

This application was prepared by Ms Oshuwa Ibhanesebhor in response to a request by the Expert Committee for a review of the role of codeine and/or loperamide in the treatment of symptomatic diarrhoea in adults. Expert reviews were prepared by Professor Abdol Majid Cheraghali and Professor Jennifer Welbeck.

In 2005, an application for the deletion of codeine was considered by the Expert Committee. A review prepared by the International Society of Drug

Bulletins (ISDB) showed that there was no high-quality evidence to support efficacy of codeine in the treatment of diarrhoea. It was retained on the Model List at that time based on the need for a treatment for symptomatic diarrhoea in adults with certain conditions, such as HIV/AIDS.

The application provided safety and efficacy data for both codeine phosphate and/or loperamide compared with other treatments or placebo. There were 17 RCTs for the treatment of acute, chronic or chemotherapy-induced diarrhoea but only 1 of these included codeine (*317–333*). All the studies reported at least one clinically relevant outcome but the majority of the studies had serious methodological flaws and a high risk of bias. When compared to placebo, loperamide improved control of diarrhoea, in both acute and chronic diarrhoea, although the results were not considered clinically significant (*318-321*). None of the studies reported any serious adverse events associated with the use of loperamide; the most commonly reported adverse effects were nausea, abdominal pain, and constipation. No studies were identified comparing loperamide with codeine phosphate for the treatment of acute diarrhoea. Loperamide was not found to be as effective as octreotide in the treatment of chemotherapy-induced diarrhoea (*322, 323*). The Committee also noted that no studies were found that evaluated the effectiveness of loperamide or codeine phosphate for the treatment of diarrhoea in people with HIV/AIDS.

The Committee did not recommend the inclusion of loperamide on the WHO Model List, due to the lack of high-quality evidence of efficacy for the use of loperamide in the treatment of acute or chronic diarrhoea in adults and the lack of evidence that loperamide is effective and safe in the treatment of diarrhoea in people with HIV/AIDS or for the treatment of chemotherapy-induced diarrhoea.

Based on the findings of the previous ISDB review of codeine phosphate and the lack of new evidence presented in the current application to support the use of codeine phosphate in the treatment of symptomatic diarrhoea in adults, the Committee recommended that it should be deleted from the Model List. The Committee also recommended that the section heading be deleted.

Section 18: Hormones, other endocrine medicines and contraceptives

Section 18.4: Estrogens

Ethinylestradiol (deletion)

Section 18.7: Progestogens

Norethisterone and medroxyprogesterone acetate (deletion)

In 2003, the Expert Committee raised a question about the public health relevance of continuing to include medroxyprogesterone acetate (MPA) on the EML for hormone replacement therapy (HRT). In 2005 this was extended to include uncertainty of the need for ethinylestradiol and also norethisterone. The Secretariat has therefore commissioned reviews of all three products for the current meeting. They were added to the List in 1979 for use in HRT and although the safety of medroxyprogesterone acetate has been subsequently evaluated, the efficacy and safety of all three medicines for HRT have not been reassessed since the publication of the large studies of HRT demonstrating no cardiovascular benefit as well as the increased risk of breast cancer. WHO therefore commissioned reviews from the University of Split as a branch of the Italian Cochrane Centre.

Expert reviews were provided by Professor Hany Abdel-Aleem, Dr Lenita Wannmacher, and Professor Jennifer Welbeck. The Department of Reproductive Health Research, WHO, recommends retention of MPA for HRT and deletion of ethinylestradiol and norethisterone.

The reviews provide a comprehensive literature search for each medicine in relation to potential benefits of HRT, in terms of symptomatic relief and effects on surrogate markers. For ethinylestradiol, the review includes also a RCT and systematic review (*334*), showing effects on bone density that were used as the basis of the claim for reduction in postmenopausal osteoporosis.

For MPA, the reviews cite the studies measuring effect on bleeding patterns, bone density, lipid concentrations, mammographic findings, cardiovascular effects, menopausal symptoms, metabolism, overall efficacy and safety as well as 'other effects'.

For norethisterone, the review presents a systematic review and 3 RCTs of use of norethisterone as HRT, and 8 systematic reviews and 10 RCTs for use in the treatment of dysfunctional uterine bleeding. Norethisterone was generally less effective than alternatives for the latter indication.

The reviews do not provide any information about the potential harms of HRT. The main risks that have been identified are the increased risk of breast cancer (from the Million Women Study; *335*), RR for current users 1.66 (95% CI 1.58–1.75), and the increased risk of thromboembolic events (*336*): pooled RR 2.15 (95% CI 1.61–2.86), pulmonary embolus RR 2.15 (95% CI 1.41–3.28), and stroke RR 1.44 (95% CI 1.10–1.89). There is also no evidence to support reduction in risk of cardiovascular disease (*337*) – one of the main claims for HRT – and the evidence for reduction in fractures is limited to change in bone mineral density, an uncertain surrogate. However, there is continuing controversy about the overall risk benefit balance.

Most guidelines today recommend HRT for short-term use only, for symptom relief. WHO does not have a treatment guideline for menopausal symptoms. The benefits and risks of use of HRT have to be assessed on a case-by-case basis. There is still considerable uncertainty about the optimal short-term symptomatic management of menopause. While there are options for the management of vasomotor effects, including clonidine, there are questions about the safest and most effective way to use hormonal preparations to manage urogenital symptoms.

No comparative cost information was provided.

The Committee noted that long-term hormone replacement treatment of menopause is no longer considered appropriate, notwithstanding individuals' possible need for treatment of symptoms. The Committee therefore decided to delete all three medicines for this indication, but to signal the need for a review of the short-term symptomatic management of menopause and the development of guidelines in this regard. For this reason, the section subheading would be retained until a proposal for inclusion of an alternative estrogen is received and reviewed. However, as progestins are needed for the management of dysfunctional uterine bleeding, MPA was retained, with a square box symbol, in the 5 mg oral solid dosage form, for this purpose. This would allow for the procurement of norethisterone in settings where this is the only product available.

Section 18.5: Insulins and other antidiabetic agents

Glucagon (inclusion)

An application was prepared by Daniel Agarwal, Dorothy Chyung, Brittany Carson, Lina Yi, Lena Makaroun, Rosa Kim, Sandeep Kishore, and Professor Marcus Reidenberg, Weill Cornell Medical College, New York, USA, for the inclusion of glucagon on the Model List. Listing was requested as an individual medicine.

Expert reviews were prepared by Dr Lenita Wannmacher and Professor David Ofori-Adjei. Comments were received from Dr Shanti Mendis, Coordinator, Chronic Diseases Prevention and Management, WHO.

The application provided evidence that hypoglycaemia is a common cause for admission to hospital for both adults and children in low-, middle-, and high-income settings (*338–341*) and the prevalence of hypoglycaemia in paediatric emergency presentations is up to 7.3% (*342–344*).

The results of three studies (*345–347*) were provided to support the efficacy and safety of glucagon for the treatment of hypoglycaemia. The Committee noted that there were no RCTs comparing glucagon to alternative treatments for the management of hypoglycaemia. Glucagon appears to be well tolerated and can be used for the management of hypoglycaemia in adults, children, and pregnant women, however no evidence was identified for its use in neonates. The Committee also noted that glucagon has the advantage over 25% and 50% dextrose solutions as it can be given subcutaneously or intramuscularly, as well as in non-hospital settings for the treatment of hypoglycaemia in patients unable to ingest oral glucose due to impaired consciousness. The Committee noted that the cost of recombinant glucagon injection 1 mg/ml appears to be generally higher than 500 ml of 5% dextrose, but the price varies widely.

The Committee concluded that the use of glucagon to treat hypoglycaemia is unlikely to be assessed in high-quality trials in the future, because it is relatively well established as a treatment in high-income countries and it is hard to define what type of comparative trial could be approved ethically. Based on public health need, evidence of safety and efficacy, and the fact that inclusion in the Model List might push prices down, the Committee decided to add glucagon to the EML and the EMLc. The Committee particularly noted the increasing number of patients in developing countries needing treatment with insulin and the concerted efforts to improve access to such treatment in resource-constrained settings. The Committee therefore saw glucagon as a necessary adjunct to this effort, but recommended that careful attention be paid to the acquisition costs. The Secretariat was asked to amend the subheadings of the Lists accordingly.

Review of the evidence comparing insulin (human or animal) with analogue insulins (review)

As part of the development of WHO advice concerning noncommunicable diseases (for the United Nations summit in September 2011) and diabetes in particular, questions have been raised by low- and middle-income countries about the role of insulin analogues compared to standard recombinant human insulin. The main concern is whether insulin analogues are cost effective or affordable, compared to recombinant human insulin. Some countries are spending significant proportions of the pharmaceutical budget on analogue insulins and at the same time, there are problems with lack of availability of standard recombinant human insulin. Insulins derived from animals are no longer available in most markets. The Secretariat has therefore commissioned a review, prepared by Ms Patti Whyte, of the comparative effectiveness and cost–effectiveness of analogue insulins compared to recombinant human insulin. The products considered are: insulin glargine, insulin detemir, insulin aspart, insulin lispro, and insulin glulisine. Expert reviews were provided by Professor Noël Cranswick and Professor Rohini Fernandopulle.

The review updates a published systematic review (*348*). An additional 35 published trials were identified, 8 of which could be included in an updated meta-analysis. Populations covered in the review include both adults and children with type 1 diabetes and adults with type 2 diabetes. Most studies were carried out in high-income country settings. The outcomes evaluated were standard surrogates for diabetic control (change in HbA1c), severe hypoglycaemic episodes or nocturnal hypoglycaemic episodes, and the risk of malignancy.

While many of the comparisons show a statistically significant difference between analogue insulin and standard recombinant human insulin, there is no evidence of a clinically significant difference in most outcomes for the majority of the studies. The Committee noted that the overall quality of evidence is low or of very-low quality for all outcomes for all comparisons. The reasons for downgrading the quality of evidence include limitations in the design of the studies, the potential for reporting bias as well as some inconsistency of results.

Comparative cost data were evaluated. The cost–effectiveness estimates vary widely, from €500/QALY to £412 000/QALY, due to very uncertain estimates of the clinical effect as well as variation in costs and resources used in the different models.

The Committee considered that the insulin analogues currently offer no clinical advantage over recombinant human insulin and there is still concern about possible long-term adverse effects.

Section 22: Oxytocics and anti-oxytocics

Section 22.1: Oxytocics

Misoprostol (new formulation)

In 2009 the Expert Committee reviewed an application for the addition of misoprostol for the prevention of postpartum haemorrhage (PPH). The application was rejected due to insufficient evidence of efficacy compared to placebo, evidence of a significant risk of shivering and fever, and concerns about possible increased mortality. The Committee requested in 2009 that a review of the safety of misoprostol should be undertaken and that data from ongoing trials in community settings should be presented in subsequent applications.

An updated application for the inclusion of misoprostol 100-microgram and 200-microgram tablets has been submitted by Gynuity Health Projects and Venture Strategies Innovations for the prevention and treatment of postpartum haemorrhage. Listing is requested as an individual medicine. A review of the safety of misoprostol for obstetric indications, commissioned by the WHO Department of Reproductive Health Research, was prepared by Dr Lenita Wannmacher.

Expert reviews were prepared by Professor David Ofori-Adjei and Professor Hany Abdel-Aleem. Comments were received from the Departments of Reproductive Health Research and Making Pregnancy Safer; Professor Anthony J Smith, Australia; Dr Edgard Narvàez Delgardo, Nicaragua; Dr Olewale Oyeneyin, Nigeria; Dr Rosana Pellizzari, Canada; Dr Amanuel Gessessew, Ethiopia; Reproductive Health Technologies Project, Washington, USA; Maternal Life International, USA; American Association of Pro-life Obstetricians and Gynecologists; and Médecins Sans Frontières. The WHO Departments of

Reproductive Health Research and Making Pregnancy Safer provided comments on both applications.

Misoprostol is currently included on the EML as:

- a 25-microgram vaginal tablet, for use in induction of labour, on the Complementary List (added in 2005);
- a 200-microgram tablet in combination with mifepristone, for termination of pregnancy (where legally permitted and culturally acceptable), on the Complementary List (added in 2005); and
- a 200-microgram tablet for the management of incomplete abortion and miscarriage, on the Complementary List (added 2009).

The Committee noted that updated WHO guidelines (*349*, *350*) and other international guidelines (*351–353*) recommend misoprostol for the prevention and treatment of PPH due to atony, in situations where parenteral uterotonics are not available. Where oxytocin is available, it is more effective and cheaper than misoprostol and is therefore the recommended treatment.

Prevention of postpartum haemorrhage

The application provided the results from four RCTs (*354–357*) to support the use of misoprostol for the prevention of PPH in settings where injectable uterotonics are not available or feasible to use. The Committee noted that the results of three of the four studies were available at the time of the last Expert Committee meeting in 2009 (*354–356*) but additional data are now available from a recently completed study from Pakistan (*357*). All four studies were undertaken in community settings, but only two studies (*356*, *357*) evaluated orally-administered 600 micrograms misoprostol or placebo when administered by non-skilled providers. The most favourable results were from the Derman study (*356*), with estimates of relative risks of 0.53 (95% CI 0.39–0.74) and 0.20 (95% CI 0.04–0.91) for prevention of moderate and severe PPH, respectively. Results from the new study (*357*) suggest there may be a benefit from use of misoprostol by traditional birth attendants or assistants provided with training on the use of the product at home deliveries; relative risks for prevention of moderate and severe PPH were 0.76 (95% CI 0.59–0.97) and 0.57 (95% CI 0.27–1.22), respectively. The Committee noted that no maternal deaths were reported and rates of referral to a higher level of care were similar in the two groups.

Treatment of postpartum haemorrhage

The Committee evaluated the results from two high-quality RCTs (*358*, *359*) comparing misoprostol 800 micrograms sublingually with oxytocin 40 IU for the treatment of PPH in a hospital setting. The Committee noted that in women with excessive postpartum bleeding suspected to be due to uterine atony, who had received prophylactic oxytocin during the third stage of labour, the use of misoprostol was non-inferior to additional oxytocin (*358*). In the most recent study, in women with PPH, who had not received prophylactic oxytocin, misoprostol was inferior to oxytocin (*359*).

Safety in prevention and treatment of PPH

With regard to safety, the most common side-effects associated with the postpartum administration of misoprostol are shivering and pyrexia (*360*). Studies show the rates of shivering and fever to be related, and to be dose- and route-dependent (*360–362*). A 2007 Cochrane Review found an increase in the rate of fever following postpartum administration of 600 micrograms compared with 400 micrograms (17% versus 8%, respectively; RR 2.12; 95% CI 1.44–3.12) (*363*). Compared to placebo, a recent meta-analysis shows that the risk of pyrexia is increased threefold with 400 micrograms misoprostol and sixfold with 600 micrograms misoprostol when administered during the third stage of labour (*364*). Higher rates of shivering and elevated body temperature are also associated with oral and sublingual routes of administration. Shivering following misoprostol administration was reported among 52% of women in India, and 10% in Pakistan (*356*, *357*). In comparison, the rates of shivering in the control arms of these studies (placebo in India and Pakistan trials) averaged 12%. Reports of fever following misoprostol administration were infrequent in these studies. In the India and Pakistan trials, fever was reported among 4% and 1% of women given misoprostol, respectively. Rates of fever were comparably low in the control arms. Misoprostol use was not associated with increased rates of nausea, vomiting, or diarrhoea during the third stage of labour in these trials. Furthermore, there was no evidence of adverse effects on neonates among mothers given misoprostol in India (*356*).

The two studies in the treatment trials testing an 800-microgram dose of sublingual misoprostol for PPH treatment documented rates of shivering that range from 37% to 47%, compared with a 15% rate of shivering among women given treatment with IV oxytocin (*359*, *365*). Rates of fever after treatment were also more common in the misoprostol group (34% versus 10%, respectively) (*359*, *365*).

Dose and route of administration

The Committee noted that there is some evidence that 600 micrograms given orally is effective and safe for the *prevention* of PPH in settings where parenteral uterotonics are not available or feasible. From the trials provided of *treatment* of PPH, 800 micrograms sublingual misoprostol is inferior to oxytocin as first-line treatment and at best, non-inferior to oxytocin when used as supplementary treatment in non-responsive women. In addition, there is no evidence to support the safety and efficacy of the 800-microgram dose for treatment of PPH when given to women who have previously received prophylactic misoprostol 600 micrograms orally.

There is still some uncertainty regarding the most effective dose and route of administration for the prevention and treatment of PPH.

Recommendations

Prevention:

After consideration of the evidence for efficacy and safety, the Committee decided to add misoprostol to the EML, for the prevention of PPH in settings where parenteral uterotonics are not available or feasible. The Committee decided to amend the note to read as follows: "For the management of incomplete abortion and miscarriage, and for the prevention of postpartum haemorrhage where oxytocin is not available or cannot be safely used". In addition, the listing should be moved from the Complementary to the Core List. A note would also be added in respect to the 25-microgram vaginal tablet, as follows: "Only for use for induction of labour where appropriate facilities are available". It was noted that the dose required for prevention (600 micrograms) could be achieved with the 200-microgram presentation and therefore the 100-microgram presentation was not included.

Treatment:

For the use of 800 micrograms misoprostol sublingually as a first-line treatment of PPH, the benefit–risk ratio is in favour of oxytocin use as a first-line treatment. In addition, there is no evidence to support the safety of an 800-microgram dose of misoprostol for treatment of PPH when given to women who have previously received prophylactic misoprostol 600 micrograms orally. To recommend misoprostol for prevention and treatment of PPH could divert the attention from or reduce attempts to implement oxytocin availability, a superior treatment. For these reasons, the Committee chose not to list treatment of PPH in the note to this inclusion in the EML.

Oxytocin (change of formulation)

A request was submitted by the Department of Child and Adolescent Health and the Department of Making Pregnancy Safer to delete the term "ampoule" from the right-hand column of the listing for oxytocin to encourage the wider availability of alternative formulations of oxytocin, such as single use compact pre-filled autodisposable devices.

Expert reviews were prepared by Professor Hany Abdel-Aleem and Professor David Ofori-Adjei. Comments were received from the Program for

Appropriate Technology in Health (PATH), the developer of the Uniject™ device for oxytocin.

The Committee noted that the efficacy and safety of oxytocin is well known and that it is the recommended first-line intervention for the prevention and treatment of PPH. The Committee noted that PATH has developed a Uniject device, which holds a prefilled dose of 1.0 ml (10 IU) oxytocin in a disposable, cushion-like package with a sterile needle attached. This product has been registered in several South American countries and in India and its acceptability and feasibility have been evaluated in field trials in several resource-poor settings (*366–369*). Given the risks associated with unsafe injections (*370*, *371*), the Uniject device may help reduce the risk of transmission of bloodborne pathogens.

The Committee recommended that the term "ampoule" be deleted from the right-hand column of the listing for oxytocin, to allow consideration of alterative oxytocin presentations. The listing would not preclude procurement of any particular presentation of injectable oxytocin.

Section 24: Psychotherapeutic medicines

Psychotherapeutic medicines (review of section headings)

An application was submitted by the WHO Department of Mental Health to change the structure and headings of Section 24 Psychotherapeutic medicines.

An expert review was prepared by Professor Rohini Fernandopulle.

Based on the recommendations of the WHO Department of Mental Health, the Committee supported the following changes to Section 24 in order to increase clarity and specificity of the medicines listed in this section and to make the Model List more practical for end-users:

- Change "Psychotherapeutic medicines" to "Medicines for mental and behavioural disorders" to increase clarity and specificity and to align more closely to the International Classification of Diseases (ICD)-10.
- Omit panic attacks from "Medicines used for obsessive compulsive disorder and panic attacks".
- Create a new heading "Medicines for anxiety disorders" and not have subheadings in this section, pending the completion of the Diagnostic and Statistical Manual of Mental Disorders (DSM)-5.
- Change "Medicines used in substance dependence programmes" to "Medicines for disorders due to psychoactive substance use" because the reference to substance dependence programmes is no longer appropriate following the addition of Nicotine Replacement Therapy to this category in 2009. The Committee noted that nicotine has been classified as a psychoactive substance in many scientific publications and therefore fits with the proposed classification.

Section 25: Medicines acting on the respiratory tract

Section 25.1: Anti-asthmatic medicines and medicines for chronic obstructive pulmonary disease

Salbutamol (deletion)

The Committee received a review on the proposed deletion of oral forms of salbutamol. The application was prepared by Dr Shalini Sri Ranganathan (Colombo, Sri Lanka).

An expert review was provided by Professor Anita Zaidi. Comments were also provided by Dr Shanthi Mendis, Coordinator, Chronic Diseases Prevention and Management.

The Committee had reviewed the use of oral forms salbutamol in 2009 and had concluded that (1) the inhaled route offers direct delivery to affected tissues and has a quicker onset of action and (2) inhaled salbutamol is effective in smaller doses than oral salbutamol and causes fewer adverse effects. However, it was decided to retain the oral forms with a note stating that such forms should only be used when inhaled treatment is not feasible.

The application focused on affordability of inhaled salbutamol and there were few new clinical data. Five trials and studies that compared oral and inhaled forms date from the 1970s and 1980s. All but one concluded to greater efficacy of the inhaled forms over the oral forms, while acknowledging superiority of oral forms over placebo. Similar efficacy between inhaled and oral forms required higher doses of oral salbutamol, leading to more adverse effects such as tachycardia, decreased oxygen saturation, flushing, hyperactivity, prolonged cough, and tremors. Adverse effects were dose dependent and dose limiting.

All current guidelines recommend inhaled salbutamol (symptom reliever) e.g. the Global Initiative on Asthma (GINA), NICE, SIGN (British Thoracic Society), the US Expert Panel Report 3 for the National Asthma Education and Prevention Program (NAEPP), and Australia, India, and Sri Lanka guidelines (*372–380*). Two guidelines mention that where inhaled salbutamol is not available, oral forms of salbutamol can be used; but all guidelines recommend the use of inhaled salbutamol as first or only choice. Inhaled salbutamol for symptom relief must be combined with anti-inflammatory treatment, either oral leukotriene antagonists, and/or inhaled steroids (systemically in severe forms) depending on the severity of asthma, to prevent complications and reduce exacerbation frequency or duration.

The Committee reviewed other indications for oral salbutamol. The application includes a selected review of three RCTs and two systematic reviews in children with wheezing and acute respiratory infections. Two trials in India and in Canada showed no difference between salbutamol and placebo for efficacy, but more adverse effects with oral short acting beta-agonists (*381*, *382*), and a small third trial in Turkey showed that salbutamol brought no benefit over placebo in terms of hospitalization (*383*). Two systematic reviews concluded that bronchodilators were not effective and could not be recommended for routine use in the treatment of bronchiolitis and there was no benefit in bronchitis, with no effect on cough (*384*, *385*).

The Committee acknowledged that salbutamol inhalation via a metered dose inhaler requires technical training to ensure proper use and hand-breathing coordination. In infants and children, the use of a spacer is recommended.

The Committee reviewed availability and cost data but noted that there are no direct comparative data of inhaled and oral forms of salbutamol. A bottle of salbutamol syrup covers only about 5 days of treatment whereas an inhaler delivers about 200 doses, corresponding to about 60 days of treatment and the immediate costs are higher for inhalers. The Committee however considered that short-term use is not in line with effective use of salbutamol in asthma, and that over the long term, inhalers might be more cost effective.

The Committee acknowledged that inhalers and spacers may not be available in resource-poor countries. This was based on data from 14 medical stores of central Africa showing availability of inhalers in 8/14 and of spacers in 1/14, and a higher price in the private sector (US$ 2.07–7.47) than in the public sector (US$ 1.30–7.25) (*386*). Similarly a survey in India found that inhalers were available in the public sector of 1/5 states and in only 2/20 public health facilities in that state, but cost was not an issue as medicines were delivered free of charge in the public sector. Availability was greater in the private sector (83–100%) and inhalers were available in all 5 states at about 0.86 to 0.96 times the international recommended price. A month's treatment of inhaled beclomethasone and salbutamol would represent about 2 days' wages of an unskilled government worker (*387*). The Committee noted the report on the availability of essential asthma medicines in 36 countries which concluded that availability varies 14–88.4% in the public sector and 47–79% in the private sector (*388*). The Committee also noted unpublished data showing that inhalers were available in only 3/8 teaching hospitals, but in 96% of private sector pharmacies in Sri Lanka.

The Committee acknowledged the affordability issue of salbutamol inhalers, but considered that oral salbutamol represents insufficient and inappropriate management of asthma and therefore recommended that oral salbutamol be deleted from the EML, with inclusion of a note to the effect that oral dosage forms only be considered in the absence of inhaled alternatives or the means to use them safely and effectively in the management of asthma.

New section: Haemaglobinopathies

Hydroxycarbamide (inclusion)

A proposal for inclusion of a new section of the List, covering medicines for sickle-cell disease, was submitted to the Expert Committee by Professor Kathleen A. Neville, Associate Professor of Pediatrics, University of Missouri, Kansas City, USA and Professor Julie A. Panepinto, Department of Pediatrics, The Children's Research Institute of the Children's Hospital of Wisconsin, Milwaukee, USA.

Expert reviews were prepared by Dr Kalle Hoppu and Professor Noël Cranswick.

The Committee recognized that sickle-cell disease (SCD) is an important public health problem in many parts of the world. The Committee noted that treatment with hydroxycarbamide can significantly decrease the incidence of painful crises and can be effective in the treatment of acute chest syndrome, priapism, and in reducing overall mortality in adult patients (*389*, *390*). The Committee noted that evidence from a systematic review (*391*) supported the safety and efficacy of hydroxycarbamide for the treatment of SCD in children aged 1 to 14 years.

The Committee noted that although hydroxycarbamide is potentially mutagenic and carcinogenic, there are no definitive data to suggest that the incidence of malignancy is increased in adult SCD patients who receive hydroxycarbamide. The Committee concluded that the risk of death due to SCD-related complications is greater than the potential for hydroxycarbamide induced leukaemia in adults.

The Committee noted that there are no evidence-based guidelines for the treatment of SCD-associated acute pain episodes, but the commonly used medicines for pain management included NSAIMs, such as ibuprofen, paracetamol, and morphine and these are already included in the WHO Model List. Deferoxamine is used to treat iron overload resulting from chronic red blood cell infusion in SCD patients with acute chest syndrome, refractory pain, or following a stroke and is already listed on the current Model List. Deferoxamine would be added under this new section, with a note about oral alternatives (see pages 21–23).

The Committee noted that prophylactic penicillin is recommended for the prevention of infections by *S. pneumoniae* in children with SCD (*392*) and that pneumococcal vaccination should be given to children with SCD to reduce the risk of bacteraemia with *S. pneumoniae*. Penicillin and pneumococcal vaccine are both listed in the current EML.

Although the Committee expressed concern about the addition of a new section specifically for sickle-cell disease, it was concerned about this selection being less visible if listed in Section 8.2 Cytotoxic medicines. The Committee therefore decided to add a subsection under Section 10, as 10.3 Other medicines for haemoglobinopathies and to list hydroxycarbamide for adults and children, based on the evidence of its safety and efficacy. Hydroxycarbamide would be added to the Complementary List.

7. Summary of recommendations

17th WHO Model List of Essential Medicines

Additions to Model List

Section 1.1. General anaesthetics and oxygen was subdivided into Section 1.1.1 Inhalational medicines and Section 1.1.2. Injectable medicines. Section 1.1.1. Isoflurane inhalation was added because it causes less hepatic failure than halothane and has advantages for maintenance of anaesthesia.

Section 1.1.2. Propofol injection: 10 mg/ml; 20 mg/ml was added because there is high-quality evidence showing that it is as safe and effective as thiopental. A note was added to indicate that thiopental could be used as an alternative depending on local availability and cost.

Section 1.3. Midazolam injection: 1 mg/ml; tablet: 7.5 mg; 15 mg was added with a square box to the Core List, replacing diazepam, due to a large body of evidence to support its safety and efficacy, its wide availability, and relatively low cost.

Section 4.2. Succimer oral solid dosage form: 100 mg added to the Complementary List based on evidence of short-term efficacy, its favourable safety profile compared to other antidotes for lead poisoning, and the potential for cost savings because it can be administered orally and does not require hospitalization unlike parenteral antidotes.

Section 6.1.2. Albendazole tablet (chewable) 400 mg was added based on evidence of efficacy and safety for the treatment of filariasis in combination with ivermectin.

Section 6.2.2. Clarithromycin tablet: 500 mg was added due to evidence of effectiveness for eradication of *H. pylori* in adults, with a note specifying for use in combination regimens for eradication of *H. pylori* in adults. Sulfamethoxazole + trimethoprim fixed-dose combination tablet: 800 mg + 160 mg was added, based on evidence of safety and efficacy for the prevention of *Pneumocystis jiroveci* in adults living with HIV.

Section 6.5.2. Miltefosine solid oral dosage form: 10 mg; 50 mg was added based on efficacy and safety in the treatment of visceral leishmaniasis in both adults and children, and evidence of safety and efficacy in adults with cutaneous or mucosal leishmaniasis.

Section 6.5.3. Artesunate + amodiaquine tablet: 25 mg + 67.5 mg; 50 mg + 135 mg; 100 mg + 270 mg were added due to evidence of safety and efficacy for the treatment of malaria in adults and children, with a note specifying that appropriate doses may also be achievable using combinations of the monocomponent products, including as co-blistered presentations.

Section 8.2. Paclitaxel injection: 6 mg/ml and docetaxel injection 20 mg/ml; 40 mg/ml were added, due to comparable effectiveness and safety for the treatment of early and advanced breast cancer.

Section 10.2. Tranexamic acid injection: 100 mg/ml was added due to evidence of efficacy and safety for the treatment of adult patients with trauma and significant risk of ongoing haemorrhage.

New subsection added: Section 10.3. Other medicines for haemoglobinopathies.

Section 10.3. Hydroxycarbamide tablet: 200 mg; 500 mg; 1 g was added to the Complementary List due to evidence of effectiveness for the treatment of painful crises due to sickle-cell disease in adults and children. Deferoxamine injection: 500 mg was added to this section due to its role in the treatment of iron overload resulting from chronic red blood cell infusion in patients with sickle-cell disease, with a note specifying that oral iron chelators, such as deferasirox, may be an alternative depending on cost and availability.

Section 12. Bisoprolol tablet: 1.25 mg; 5 mg replaced atenolol as the representative beta-blocker in subsections 12.1, 12.2, 12.3, due to evidence of safety and efficacy for the treatment of angina, arrhythmias and hypertension as well as concerns about the safety of atenolol, especially in older hypertensive patients. Bisoprolol tablet: 1.25 mg; 10 mg was added to subsection 12.4 with a square box, based on evidence of safety, efficacy, and cost–effectiveness for the treatment of heart failure. A note was added to all subsections specifying that metoprolol and carvedilol are the alternatives.

Section 13.1. Terbinafine cream: 1% or ointment: 1% terbinafine hydrochloride was added, due to its increasing availability from generic sources.

Section 13.2. Mupirocin cream or ointment: 2% was added, due to evidence of efficacy and safety as a topical treatment for superficial bacterial infections and the fact that inclusion in the Model List may push prices down.

Section 18.5. Glucagon injection: 1 mg/ml was added based on public health need, evidence of safety and efficacy, and the fact that inclusion in the Model List may push prices down.

Section 20. Atracurium injection: 10 mg/ml was added due to its comparative effectiveness and safety profile, current availability and lower cost than alternatives.

Section 22.1. Misoprostol tablet: 200 micrograms was added, based on evidence of safety and efficacy for the prevention of postpartum haemorrhage, where oxytocin is not available or cannot be safely used. Misoprostol tablet: 200 micrograms; vaginal tablet: 25 micrograms, moved from the

Complementary to the Core List. The note for 200-microgram tablet amended to specify it is for management of incomplete abortion and miscarriage and for prevention of postpartum haemorrhage where oxytocin is not available or cannot be used safely.

Deletions from Model List

Section 1.1.1. Square box deleted from halothane to indicate that it is no longer the representative inhalational agent.

Section 1.3.
Diazepam replaced by midazolam due to evidence indicating that diazepam, while as efficacious as midazolam, is associated with lower patient satisfaction and amnesic effect.

Promethazine oral liquid 5 mg/ml deleted due to evidence showing that it is inferior to midazolam for preoperative medication and sedation for short-term procedures.

Section 4.2. DL-methionine powder for injection: 500 mg; tablet 250 mg was deleted because of reported limited availability, the unknown real cost difference between DL-methionine and N-acetylcysteine and the fact that N-acetylcysteine has become the standard of care globally.

Section 6.1.1. Square box deleted from mebendazole because all the other benzimidazoles are already included in the Model List as individual entries.

Section 6.1.2. Suramin sodium powder for injection 1 g was deleted because it is no longer used for the treatment of filariasis.

Section 6.5.3.1. Note specifying that amodiaquine alone can be used for the treatment of *P. vivax*, *P. ovale*, and *P. malariae* was deleted. Amodiaquine should be used in combination with artesunate 50 mg.

Section 13.1. Benzoic acid + salicylic acid cream or ointment: 6% + 3% was deleted due to the addition of terbinafine cream: 1% or ointment: 1% terbinafine hydrochloride; selenium sulfide detergent-based suspension: 2% was moved from the Complementary to the Core List.

Section 13.2. Methylrosanilinium chloride (gentian violet) aqueous solution: 0.5%; tincture: 0.5% was deleted due to evidence that it may act as a carcinogen; neomycin sulfate + bacitracin ointment: 5 mg + 250 IU was deleted due to the addition of a safer and more effective alternative to the Model List.

Section 13.4. Aluminium diacetate solution: 5% was deleted due to evidence of lack of efficacy and public health need and because it can be an irritant. Section 13.4. Astringent medicines was deleted and the subsequent subsections were renumbered accordingly.

Section 17.1. Aluminium hydroxide oral liquid: 320 mg/5 ml; magnesium hydroxide oral liquid: equivalent to 550 mg magnesium oxide/10 ml were deleted due to evidence of no benefit compared to placebo and the presence of safe and effective alternatives on the Model List for the treatment of gastro-oesophageal reflux disease and non-ulcer dyspepsia. Section 17.1 heading changed to anti-ulcer medicines.

Section 17.5.3. Codeine tablet: 30 mg was deleted due to lack of public health need and evidence of safety and efficacy for the treatment of symptomatic diarrhoea in adults. The section heading was also deleted.

Section 18.4. Ethinylestradiol tablet: 10 micrograms; 50 micrograms were deleted due to evidence that these doses are no longer recommended for use in hormone replacement therapy.

Section 18.7. Norethisterone tablet: 5 mg was deleted due to evidence that this dose is no longer recommended for use in hormone replacement therapy and evidence that it is inferior to alternatives for the treatment of dysfunctional uterine bleeding.

Section 25.1. Salbutamol oral liquid: 2 mg/5 ml; tablet 2 mg; 4 mg due to evidence that oral salbutamol is inferior in terms of safety and efficacy to inhaled salbutamol and because oral salbutamol represents insufficient and inappropriate management of asthma.

Changes to sections

Section 1.1. General anaesthetics and oxygen was subdivided into Section 1.1.1 Inhalational medicines and Section 1.1.2 Injectable medicines to improve the clarity and specificity of this section.

Section 6.1.2. Diethylcarbamazine was moved from the Complementary to the Core List because it is recommended by WHO guidelines as the medicine of choice for mass administration in onchocerciasis-free areas.

New subsection added: Section 10.3. Other medicines for haemoglobinopathies due to the inclusion on the Model List of hydroxycarbamide and deferoxamine specifically for sickle-cell disease.

Section 17.5.3. Antidiarrhoeal (symptomatic) medicines in adults was deleted due to the deletion of codeine from this section.

Section 18.5. Section heading changed to "Insulins and other medicines used for diabetes" due to the addition of glucagon to this section.

Section 18.7. Medroxyprogesterone acetate with a square box tablet: 5 mg moved from the Complementary to the Core List because its use does not require special monitoring or equipment.

Section 24. Section heading changed to "Medicines for mental and behavioural disorders" to increase clarity and specificity and to align more closely with the ICD-10.

Section 24.3. Subsection heading changed to "Medicines for anxiety disorders" to increase clarity.

Section 24.3.1. Medicines used in generalized anxiety disorders deleted. Diazepam with a square box moved to Section 24.3. Subheading deleted pending the completion of the DSM-5.

Section 24.5. Subsection heading changed to "Medicines for disorders due to psychoactive substance use" because the reference to substance dependence programmes is no longer appropriate following the addition of nicotine replacement therapy to this category in 2009.

Amended dosage strength and form

Section 13.4. Urea cream or ointment: 5% was added to enable wider dosing.

Section 22.1. The term "ampoule" was removed from the right-hand column of the listing for oxytocin to allow consideration of alternative oxytocin presentations.

Rejected applications

Section 1.1. The reinstatement of ether was rejected due to alternatives with better benefit–risk balances already on the Model List.

Section 6.2.2.
Gatifloxacin was rejected due to safety concerns, the availability of alternatives, and the likelihood that supply will be limited in the future.

Isoniazid + pyridoxine + sulfamethoxazole + trimethoprim (fixed-dose combination) was rejected because the product does not yet exist.

Section 6.4.2.2. Etravirine was rejected due to the comparatively limited efficacy and long-term safety data in adults and lack of evidence in children.

Section 6.4.2.3. Darunavir was rejected due to the comparatively limited efficacy, safety, and cost–effectiveness in both adults and children in a diversity of settings and because the optimal use of darunavir is still being defined.

Section 6.4.2.4. Raltegravir was rejected due to the comparatively limited efficacy, safety, and cost–effectiveness in both adults and children in a diversity of settings and because the optimal use of raltegravir is still being defined, as well as the best combinations of medicines for third-line regimens.

Section 6.5.3. Dihydroartemisinin + piperaquine fixed-dose combination tablets: 40 mg + 320 mg; 20 mg + 160 mg were rejected due to the lack of a comprehensive review of all existing clinical trial data, including safety data and evidence that the fixed-dose combinations when given according to the recommend regimen do not deliver target doses of the components, as noted in the WHO malaria treatment guidelines.

Section 6.5.3. Pyronaridine + artesunate fixed-dose combination tablet was rejected due to the fact the product is not yet available, there are additional clinical trial data that will become available, and there is a safety issue that needs to be resolved.

Section 17.5.3. Loperamide was rejected due to lack of high-quality evidence that it is safe and effective in the treatment of acute or chronic diarrhoea in adults and lack of evidence that it is safe and effective in the treatment of diarrhoea in people living with HIV/AIDS or for the treatment of chemotherapy-induced diarrhoea.

3rd Essential Medicines List for children

Additions to EMLc

Section 1.1. General anaesthetics and oxygen was subdivided into Section 1.1.1 Inhalational medicines and Section 1.1.2. Injectable medicines. Section 1.1.1. Isoflurane inhalation was added because it causes less hepatic failure than halothane and has advantages for maintenance of anaesthesia.

Section 1.1.2. Propofol injection: 10 mg/ml; 20 mg/ml was added because there is high-quality evidence showing that it is as safe and effective as thiopental. A note was added to indicate that thiopental could be used as an alternative depending on local availability and cost.

Section 1.3. Midazolam injection: 1 mg/ml; tablet: 7.5 mg; 15 mg was added with a square box to the Core List, replacing diazepam, due to large body of evidence to support its safety and efficacy, its wide availability, and relatively low cost.

Section 2.4. Methotrexate tablet: 2.5 mg was added to the Complementary List based on evidence of safety and efficacy in children. Hydroxychloroquine tablet: 200 mg was added to the Complementary List based on evidence of effectiveness for treatment of systemic lupus erythematosus.

Section 4.2. Succimer oral solid dosage form: 100 mg was added to the Complementary List based on evidence of short-term efficacy, its favourable safety profile compared to other antidotes for lead poisoning, and the potential for cost savings because it can be administered orally and does not require hospitalization unlike parenteral antidotes.

Section 6.1.2. Albendazole tablet (chewable) 400 mg was added based on evidence of efficacy and safety for the treatment of filariasis in combination with ivermectin.

Section 6.5.2. Miltefosine solid oral dosage form: 10 mg; 50 mg was added based on efficacy and safety in the treatment of visceral leishmaniasis in both adults and children, and evidence of safety and efficacy in adults with cutaneous or mucosal leishmaniasis.

Section 6.5.3. Artesunate + amodiaquine tablet: 25 mg + 67.5 mg; 50 mg + 135 mg; 100 mg + 270 mg were added due to evidence of safety and efficacy for the treatment of malaria in adults and children, with a note specifying that appropriate doses may also be achievable using combinations of the monocomponent products, including as co-blistered presentations.

Section 8.2. Cytotoxic medicines has been restructured to provide treatment options for acute lymphoblastic leukaemia, Wilms tumour (nephroblastoma) and Burkitt lymphoma, as well as appropriate adjuvant medicines. The majority of medicines required for these regimens were already listed in this section. New additions included mesna injection: 100 mg/ml; tablet: 400 mg; 600 mg; methylprednisolone injection: 40 mg/ml; 80 mg/ml; and thioguanine solid oral dosage form: 40 mg.

Section 8.4. Lactulose solution: 3.1–3.7 g/5 ml was added as an alternative to docusate sodium for the management of opioid-induced constipation.

Section 13.1. Terbinafine cream: 1% or ointment: 1% terbinafine hydrochloride was added, due to its increasing availability from generic sources.

Section 13.2. Mupirocin cream or ointment: 2% was added, due to evidence of efficacy and safety as a topical treatment for superficial bacterial infections and the fact that inclusion in the Model List may push prices down.

Section 18.5. Glucagon injection: 1 mg/ml was added based on public health need, evidence of safety and efficacy, and the fact that inclusion in the Model List may push prices down.

Deletions from EMLc

Section 2.2. Codeine 15 mg was deleted due to evidence indicating that its analgesic effect is low or absent in neonates and young children and evidence of considerable pharmacogenetic variability among populations, making its efficacy and safety questionable in an unpredictable proportion of the paediatric population.

Section 4.2. Penicillamine solid oral dosage form: 250 mg was deleted due to the higher risk of adverse events compared to other oral lead chelators in children.

Section 6.1.1. Square box was deleted from mebendazole because all the other benzimidazoles are already included in the Model List as individual entries.

Section 6.5.3.1. Note specifying that amodiaquine alone can be used for the treatment of *P. vivax*, *P. ovale*, and *P. malariae* was deleted. Amodiaquine should be used in combination with artesunate 50 mg.

Section 8.2. Chlorambucil, 5-fluorouracil, bleomycin, dacarbazine, procarbazine, ifosamide, and etoposide were deleted because they are not needed for the treatment protocols for acute lymphoblastic leukaemia, Wilms tumour and Burkitt lymphoma.

Section 13.1. Benzoic acid + salicylic acid cream or ointment: 6% + 3% was deleted due to the addition of terbinafine cream: 1% or ointment: 1% terbinafine hydrochloride. Selenium sulfide detergent-based suspension: 2% was moved from the Complementary to the Core List.

Section 13.2. Methylrosanilinium chloride (gentian violet) aqueous solution: 0.5%; tincture: 0.5% was deleted due to evidence that it may act as a carcinogen; neomycin sulfate + bacitracin ointment: 5 mg + 250 IU was deleted due to the addition of a safer and more effective alternative to the Model List.

Section 13.4. Aluminium diacetate solution: 5% was deleted due to evidence of lack of efficacy and public health need and because it can be an irritant. Section 13.4. Astringent medicines was deleted and the subsequent subsections were renumbered accordingly.

Section 17.1. Aluminium hydroxide oral liquid: 320 mg/5 ml; magnesium hydroxide oral liquid: equivalent to 550 mg magnesium oxide/10 ml were deleted due to evidence of no benefit compared to placebo and the presence of safe and effective alternatives on the Model List for the treatment of gastro-oesophageal reflux disease and non-ulcer dyspepsia. Section 17.1 heading changed to "Anti-ulcer medicines".

Section 25.1. Salbutamol oral liquid: 2 mg/5 ml; tablet 2 mg; 4 mg was deleted due to evidence that oral salbutamol is inferior in terms of safety and efficacy to inhaled salbutamol and because oral salbutamol represents insufficient and inappropriate management of asthma.

Changes to sections

Section 1.1. General anaesthetics and oxygen was subdivided into Section 1.1.1 Inhalational medicines and Section 1.1.2 Injectable medicines to improve the clarity and specificity of this section.

Section 6.1.2. Diethylcarbamazine was moved from the Complementary to the Core List because it is recommended by WHO guidelines as the medicine of choice for mass administration in onchocerciasis-free areas.

Section 6.5.5.1. Melarsoprol was moved to the Complementary List due to safety concerns of its use in children.

Section 8.2. Cytotoxic medicines has been restructured to provide treatment options for acute lymphoblastic leukaemia, Wilms tumour (nephroblastoma) and Burkitt lymphoma, as well as appropriate adjuvant medicines.

Section 8.3. Hormones and antihormones were deleted due to the medicines from this section being incorporated in the newly restructured Section 8.2.

Section 8.4. Medicines used in palliative care. Deletion of restriction of use of ibuprofen for bone pain; addition of ondansetron, fluoxetine, midazolam, and lactulose to this section.

New subsection added: Section 10.3. Other medicines for haemoglobinopathies due to the inclusion on the Model List of hydroxycarbamide and deferoxamine specifically for sickle-cell disease.

Section 18.5. Section heading changed to "Insulins and other medicines used for diabetes" due to addition of glucagon to this section.

Section 24. Section heading changed to "Medicines for mental and behavioural disorders" to increase clarity and specificity and to align more closely with the ICD-10.

Section 24.3. Subsection heading changed to "Medicines for anxiety disorders" to increase clarity.

Section 24.3.1. Medicines used in generalized anxiety disorders deleted. Diazepam with a square box moved to Section 24.3. Subheading deleted pending the completion of the DSM-5.

Section 24.5. Subsection heading changed to "Medicines for disorders due to psychoactive substance use" in line with the changes to the heading changes on the complete Model List.

Amended dosage strength and form

Section 2.1. Ibuprofen oral liquid: 200 mg/5 ml added as a safe alternative to paracetamol.

Section 8.4. Ibuprofen 200 mg/5 ml replaced 100 mg/ml to enable more accurate dosing in young children.

Section 13.4. Urea cream or ointment: 5% to enable wider dosing.

Section 17.5.2. Zinc sulfate solid oral dosage form: 20 mg replaced the oral liquid: 10 mg per unit dosage form and tablet: 10 mg per unit dosage form due to the much higher cost of treating children aged more than 6 months with two 10-mg tablets as opposed to one 20-mg tablet, and safety concerns regarding the administration of 20 mg to children aged less than 6 months.

Rejected medicines

Section 4.2. 2,3-dimercapto-1-propanesulfonic acid (DMPS) was rejected due to insufficient evidence of effectiveness and safety.

Section 8.2. Imatinib due to the rarity of chronic myeloid leukaemia in children, limited evidence of efficacy and long-term safety in children, and the high cost of the medicine.

Section 15. Chlorhexidine (change of formulation) was rejected due to the lack of a commercially available preparation of 7.1% chlorhexidine digluconate solution or gel delivering 4% chlorhexidine.

Recommendations for reviews

1. Should adults with rheumatoid arthritis be treated with chloroquine compared to hydroxychloroquine?
2. Should adults with lead poisoning be treated with penicillamine compared to other lead chelators?
3. Should low molecular weight heparin or an alternative be included on the EML for adults?
4. Should elderly patients with type 2 diabetes be treated with glibenclamide compared to other sulfonylureas?
5. Which long-acting muscle relaxant should be used in adults and children?
6. Should adults and children with mild to moderate acne be treated with benzoyl peroxide compared to other topical preparations for acne?
7. Should adults and children with psoriasis be treated with coal tar solution compared to other topical preparations for psoriasis?
8. Should adults and children with gastro-oesophageal reflux or non-ulcer dyspepsia be treated with H_2-antagonists compared to proton pump inhibitors?
9. Should children with *H. pylori* infection be treated with *H. pylori* eradication therapy compared to no treatment?
10. Can neonates with superficial bacterial skin infections be safely treated with mupirocin compared with other topical antibiotics, such as tetracycline?
11. Should adults and children with dengue fever be treated with intravenous colloids compared to crystalloids?
12. Should adults and children with toxic alcohol poisoning be treated with fomepizole compared to ethanol?
13. What anaesthetics can safely be used in neonates?
14. Should adults with type 2 diabetes be treated with 1) alpha-glucosidase inhibitors, such as acarbose; 2) amylin analogues, such as pramlintide; and 3) dipeptidyl peptidase-4 inhibitors such as sitagliptin and meglitinides such as repaglinide and mitiglinide compared with other classes of oral

hypoglycaemic medicines (metformin; sulfonylureas such as glibenclamide, glimepiride, and gliclazide; thiazolidinediones such as pioglitazone and rosiglitazone)?

Medicines marked for consideration of deletion at the next meeting

1. Penicillamine (adults)
2. Levamisole (adults and children)
3. Niclosamide (adults and children)
4. Dithranol (adults)
5. Ranitidine (adults and children)

Missing essential medicines

Chlorhexidine 4% solution or gel.
Isoniazid + pyridoxine + sulfamethoxazole + trimethoprim (fixed-dose combination).

Annex 1

17th WHO Model List of Essential Medicines

Explanatory Notes

The **Core List** presents a list of minimum medicine needs for a basic health-care system, listing the most efficacious, safe and cost-effective medicines for priority conditions. Priority conditions are selected on the basis of current and estimated future public health relevance, and potential for safe and cost-effective treatment.

The **Complementary List** presents essential medicines for priority diseases, for which specialized diagnostic or monitoring facilities, and/or specialist medical care, and/or specialist training are needed. In case of doubt medicines may also be listed as complementary on the basis of consistent higher costs or less attractive cost–effectiveness in a variety of settings.

The **square box symbol** (□) is primarily intended to indicate similar clinical performance within a pharmacological class. The listed medicine should be the example of the class for which there is the best evidence for effectiveness and safety. In some cases, this may be the first medicine that is licensed for marketing; in other instances, subsequently licensed compounds may be safer or more effective. Where there is no difference in terms of efficacy and safety data, the listed medicine should be the one that is generally available at the lowest price, based on international drug price information sources. Not all square boxes are applicable to medicine selection for children – see the 3rd EMLc for details.

Therapeutic equivalence is only indicated on the basis of reviews of efficacy and safety and when consistent with WHO clinical guidelines. National lists should not use a similar symbol and should be specific in their final selection, which would depend on local availability and price.

The [a] symbol indicates that there is an age or weight restriction on use of the medicine; details for each medicine can be found in Table 1.1.

Where the [c] symbol is placed next to the Complementary List it signifies that the medicine(s) require(s) specialist diagnostic or monitoring facilities, and/or specialist medical care, and/or specialist training for use in children.

Where the [c] symbol is placed next to an individual medicine or strength of medicine it signifies that there is a specific indication for restricting its use to children.

The presence of an entry on the Essential Medicines List carries no assurance as to pharmaceutical quality. It is the responsibility of the relevant national or regional drug regulatory authority to ensure that each product is of appropriate pharmaceutical quality (including stability) and that when relevant, different products are interchangeable.

For recommendations and advice concerning all aspects of the quality assurance of medicines see the WHO Medicines web site http://www.who.int/medicines/areas/quality_assurance/en/index.html.

Medicines and dosage forms are listed in alphabetical order within each section and there is no implication of preference for one form over another. Standard treatment guidelines should be consulted for information on appropriate dosage forms.

The main terms used for dosage forms in the Essential Medicines List can be found in Table 1.2.

Definitions of many of these terms and pharmaceutical quality requirements applicable to the different categories are published in the current edition of *The International Pharmacopoeia* http://www.who.int/medicines/publications/pharmacopoeia/en/index.html.

1. ANAESTHETICS

1.1 General anaesthetics and oxygen

1.1.1 *Inhalational medicines*

halothane	**Inhalation.**
isoflurane	**Inhalation.**
nitrous oxide	**Inhalation.**
oxygen	**Inhalation** (medicinal gas).

1.1.2 *Injectable medicines*

ketamine	**Injection:** 50 mg (as hydrochloride)/ml in 10-ml vial.
propofol*	**Injection:** 10 mg/ml; 20 mg/ml. * Thiopental may be used as an alternative depending on local availability and cost.

1.2 Local anaesthetics

□ bupivacaine	**Injection:** 0.25%; 0.5% (hydrochloride) in vial. **Injection for spinal anaesthesia**: 0.5% (hydrochloride) in 4-ml ampoule to be mixed with 7.5% glucose solution.
□ lidocaine	**Injection:** 1%; 2% (hydrochloride) in vial. **Injection for spinal anaesthesia:** 5% (hydrochloride) in 2-ml ampoule to be mixed with 7.5% glucose solution. **Topical forms:** 2% to 4% (hydrochloride).
lidocaine + epinephrine (adrenaline)	**Dental cartridge:** 2% (hydrochloride) + epinephrine 1:80 000. **Injection:** 1%; 2% (hydrochloride **or** sulfate) + epinephrine 1:200 000 in vial.

Complementary List

ephedrine	***Injection:*** *30 mg (hydrochloride)/ml in 1-ml ampoule.* *(For use in spinal anaesthesia during delivery, to prevent hypotension).*

1.3 Preoperative medication and sedation for short-term procedures

atropine	**Injection:** 1 mg (sulfate) in 1-ml ampoule.

1. ANAESTHETICS *(continued)*

□ midazolam	**Injection:** 1 mg/ml. **Oral liquid:** 2 mg/ml [c]. **Tablet:** 7.5 mg; 15 mg.
morphine	**Injection:** 10 mg (sulfate **or** hydrochloride) in 1-ml ampoule.

2. ANALGESICS, ANTIPYRETICS, NON-STEROIDAL ANTI-INFLAMMATORY MEDICINES (NSAIMs), MEDICINES USED TO TREAT GOUT AND DISEASE-MODIFYING AGENTS IN RHEUMATOID DISORDERS (DMARDs)

2.1 Non-opioids and non-steroidal anti-inflammatory medicines (NSAIMs)

acetylsalicylic acid	**Suppository:** 50 mg to 150 mg. **Tablet:** 100 mg to 500 mg.
ibuprofen [a]	**Oral liquid:** 200 mg/5 ml. **Tablet:** 200 mg; 400 mg. [a] >3 months.
paracetamol*	**Oral liquid:** 125 mg/5 ml. **Suppository:** 100 mg. **Tablet:** 100 mg to 500 mg. * Not recommended for anti-inflammatory use due to lack of proven benefit to that effect.

***Complementary List* [c]**

*acetylsalicylic acid**	***Suppository:** 50 mg to 150 mg.* ***Tablet:** 100 mg to 500 mg.* * *For use for rheumatic fever, juvenile arthritis, Kawasaki disease.*

2.2 Opioid analgesics

codeine*	**Tablet:** 30 mg (phosphate). * The Expert Committee has requested a review of the comparative effectiveness and safety, for possible deletion of this medicine at its next meeting.
morphine	**Injection:** 10 mg (morphine hydrochloride **or** morphine sulfate) in 1-ml ampoule. **Oral liquid:** 10 mg (morphine hydrochloride **or** morphine sulfate)/5 ml. **Tablet:** 10 mg (morphine sulfate). **Tablet (prolonged release):** 10 mg; 30 mg; 60 mg (morphine sulfate).

2. ANALGESICS, ANTIPYRETICS, NON-STEROIDAL ANTI-INFLAMMATORY MEDICINES (NSAIMs), MEDICINES USED TO TREAT GOUT AND DISEASE-MODIFYING AGENTS IN RHEUMATOID DISORDERS (DMARDs) *(continued)*

2.3 Medicines used to treat gout

allopurinol	**Tablet:** 100 mg.

2.4 Disease-modifying agents used in rheumatoid disorders (DMARDs)

chloroquine*	**Tablet:** 100 mg; 150 mg (as phosphate or sulfate). * The Expert Committee has requested a review of the comparative effectiveness and safety, for possible deletion of this medicine at its next meeting.

Complementary List

azathioprine	***Tablet:*** *50 mg.*
hydroxychloroquine [c]	***Solid oral dosage form:*** *200 mg (as sulfate).*
methotrexate	***Tablet:*** *2.5 mg (as sodium salt).*
penicillamine	***Solid oral dosage form:*** *250 mg.*
sulfasalazine	***Tablet:*** *500 mg.*

3. ANTIALLERGICS AND MEDICINES USED IN ANAPHYLAXIS

□ chlorphenamine [a]	**Injection:** 10 mg (hydrogen maleate) in 1-ml ampoule. **Oral liquid:** 2 mg/5 ml (hydrogen maleate) [c]. **Tablet:** 4 mg (hydrogen maleate). [a] >1 year.
dexamethasone	**Injection:** 4 mg/ml in 1-ml ampoule (as disodium phosphate salt).
epinephrine (adrenaline)	**Injection:** 1 mg (as hydrochloride **or** hydrogen tartrate) in 1-ml ampoule.
hydrocortisone	**Powder for injection:** 100 mg (as sodium succinate) in vial.
□ prednisolone	**Oral liquid:** 5 mg/ml [c]. **Tablet:** 5 mg; 25 mg.

4. ANTIDOTES AND OTHER SUBSTANCES USED IN POISONINGS

4.1 Non-specific

charcoal, activated	**Powder.**

4. ANTIDOTES AND OTHER SUBSTANCES USED IN POISONINGS *(continued)*

4.2 Specific

acetylcysteine	**Injection:** 200 mg/ml in 10-ml ampoule. **Oral liquid:** 10% [c]; 20% [c].
atropine	**Injection:** 1 mg (sulfate) in 1-ml ampoule.
calcium gluconate	**Injection:** 100 mg/ml in 10-ml ampoule.
methylthioninium chloride (methylene blue)	**Injection:** 10 mg/ml in 10-ml ampoule.
naloxone	**Injection:** 400 micrograms (hydrochloride) in 1-ml ampoule.
penicillamine*	**Solid oral dosage form:** 250 mg. * The Expert Committee has requested a review of the comparative effectiveness and safety, for possible deletion of this medicine at its next meeting.
potassium ferric hexacyano-ferrate(II) -$2H_20$ (Prussian blue)	**Powder for oral administration.**
sodium nitrite	**Injection:** 30 mg/ml in 10-ml ampoule.
sodium thiosulfate	**Injection:** 250 mg/ml in 50-ml ampoule.
Complementary List	
deferoxamine	***Powder for injection:** 500 mg (mesilate) in vial.*
dimercaprol	***Injection in oil:** 50 mg/ml in 2-ml ampoule.*
sodium calcium edetate	***Injection:** 200 mg/ml in 5-ml ampoule.*
succimer	***Solid oral dosage form:** 100 mg.*

5. ANTICONVULSANTS/ANTIEPILEPTICS

carbamazepine	**Oral liquid:** 100 mg/5 ml. **Tablet (chewable):** 100 mg; 200 mg. **Tablet (scored):** 100 mg; 200 mg.
diazepam	**Gel or rectal solution:** 5 mg/ml in 0.5 ml; 2-ml; 4-ml tubes.
□ lorazepam	**Parenteral formulation:** 2 mg/ml in 1-ml ampoule; 4 mg/ml in 1-ml ampoule.

5. ANTICONVULSANTS/ANTIEPILEPTICS *(continued)*

magnesium sulfate*	**Injection:** 500 mg/ml in 2-ml ampoule; 500 mg/ml in 10-ml ampoule. * For use in eclampsia and severe pre-eclampsia and not for other convulsant disorders.
phenobarbital	**Injection:** 200 mg/ml (sodium). **Oral liquid:** 15 mg/5 ml. **Tablet:** 15 mg to 100 mg.
phenytoin	**Injection:** 50 mg/ml in 5-ml vial (sodium salt). **Oral liquid:** 25 mg to 30 mg/5 ml.* **Solid oral dosage form:** 25 mg; 50 mg; 100 mg (sodium salt). **Tablet (chewable):** 50 mg. * The presence of both 25 mg/5 ml and 30 mg/5 ml strengths on the same market would cause confusion in prescribing and dispensing and should be avoided.
valproic acid (sodium valproate)	**Oral liquid:** 200 mg/5 ml. **Tablet (crushable):** 100 mg. **Tablet (enteric-coated):** 200 mg; 500 mg (sodium valproate).
Complementary List	
ethosuximide	***Capsule:*** 250 mg. ***Oral liquid:*** 250 mg/5 ml.

6. ANTI-INFECTIVE MEDICINES

6.1 Anthelminthics

6.1.1 *Intestinal anthelminthics*

albendazole	**Tablet (chewable):** 400 mg.
levamisole*	**Tablet:** 50 mg; 150 mg (as hydrochloride). * The Expert Committee recommended that this medicine be reviewed for deletion at its next meeting. Should be used in combination with other anthelminthics.
mebendazole	**Tablet (chewable):** 100 mg; 500 mg.
niclosamide*	**Tablet (chewable):** 500 mg. * Niclosamide is listed for use when praziquantel treatment fails. The Expert Committee recommended that this medicine be reviewed for deletion at its next meeting.

6. ANTI-INFECTIVE MEDICINES *(continued)*	
praziquantel	**Tablet:** 150 mg; 600 mg.
pyrantel	**Oral liquid:** 50 mg (as embonate **or** pamoate)/ml. **Tablet (chewable):** 250 mg (as embonate **or** pamoate).
6.1.2 *Antifilarials*	
albendazole	**Tablet (chewable):** 400 mg.
diethylcarbamazine	**Tablet:** 50 mg; 100 mg (dihydrogen citrate).
ivermectin	**Tablet (scored):** 3 mg; 6 mg.
6.1.3 *Antischistosomals and other antitrematode medicines*	
praziquantel	**Tablet:** 600 mg.
triclabendazole	**Tablet:** 250 mg.
Complementary List	
*oxamniquine**	***Capsule:*** *250 mg.* ***Oral liquid:*** *250 mg/5 ml.* * *Oxamniquine is listed for use when praziquantel treatment fails.*

6.2 Antibacterials	
6.2.1 *Beta Lactam medicines*	
amoxicillin	**Powder for oral liquid:** 125 mg (as trihydrate)/5 ml; 250 mg (as trihydrate)/5 ml [c]. **Solid oral dosage form:** 250 mg; 500 mg (as trihydrate).
amoxicillin + clavulanic acid	**Oral liquid:** 125 mg amoxicillin + 31.25 mg clavulanic acid/5 ml AND 250 mg amoxicillin + 62.5 mg clavulanic acid/5 ml [c]. **Tablet:** 500 mg (as trihydrate) + 125 mg (as potassium salt).
ampicillin	**Powder for injection:** 500 mg; 1 g (as sodium salt) in vial.
benzathine benzylpenicillin	**Powder for injection:** 900 mg benzylpenicillin (= 1.2 million IU) in 5-ml vial [c]; 1.44 g benzylpenicillin (= 2.4 million IU) in 5-ml vial.
benzylpenicillin	**Powder for injection:** 600 mg (= 1 million IU); 3 g (= 5 million IU) (sodium **or** potassium salt) in vial.

6. ANTI-INFECTIVE MEDICINES *(continued)*	
cefalexin [c]	**Powder for reconstitution with water:** 125 mg/5 ml; 250 mg/5 ml (anhydrous). **Solid oral dosage form:** 250 mg (as monohydrate).
□ cefazolin* [a]	**Powder for injection:** 1 g (as sodium salt) in vial. * For surgical prophylaxis. [a] >1 month.
cefixime*	**Capsule:** 400 mg (as trihydrate). * Only listed for single-dose treatment of uncomplicated ano-genital gonorrhoea.
ceftriaxone* [a]	**Powder for injection:** 250 mg; 1 g (as sodium salt) in vial. * Do not administer with calcium and avoid in infants with hyperbilirubinemia. [a] >41 weeks corrected gestational age.
□ cloxacillin	**Capsule:** 500 mg; 1 g (as sodium salt). **Powder for injection:** 500 mg (as sodium salt) in vial. **Powder for oral liquid:** 125 mg (as sodium salt)/ 5 ml.
phenoxymethylpenicillin	**Powder for oral liquid:** 250 mg (as potassium salt)/ 5 ml. **Tablet:** 250 mg (as potassium salt).
procaine benzylpenicillin*	**Powder for injection:** 1 g (=1 million IU); 3 g (=3 million IU) in vial. * Procaine benzylpenicillin is not recommended as first-line treatment for neonatal sepsis except in settings with high neonatal mortality, when given by trained health workers in cases where hospital care is not achievable.
Complementary List	
*cefotaxime** [c]	***Powder for injection:** 250 mg per vial (as sodium salt).* ** 3rd generation cephalosporin of choice for use in hospitalized neonates.*
ceftazidime	***Powder for injection:** 250 mg **or** 1 g (as pentahydrate) in vial.*

6. ANTI-INFECTIVE MEDICINES *(continued)*

imipenem + cilastatin**	***Powder for injection:** 250 mg (as monohydrate) + 250 mg (as sodium salt); 500 mg (as monohydrate) + 500 mg (as sodium salt) in vial.* * *Only listed for the treatment of life-threatening hospital-based infection due to suspected or proven multidrug-resistant infection.* *Meropenem is indicated for the treatment of meningitis and is licensed for use in children over the age of 3 months.*

6.2.2 *Other antibacterials*

azithromycin*	**Capsule:** 250 mg; 500 mg (anhydrous). **Oral liquid:** 200 mg/5 ml. * Only listed for single-dose treatment of genital *Chlamydia trachomatis* and of trachoma.
chloramphenicol	**Capsule:** 250 mg. **Oily suspension for injection*:** 0.5 g (as sodium succinate)/ml in 2-ml ampoule. * Only for the presumptive treatment of epidemic meningitis in children older than 2 years. **Oral liquid:** 150 mg (as palmitate)/5 ml. **Powder for injection:** 1 g (sodium succinate) in vial.
□ ciprofloxacin*	**Oral liquid:** 250 mg/5 ml (anhydrous) [c]. **Solution for IV infusion:** 2 mg/ml (as hyclate) [c]. **Tablet:** 250 mg (as hydrochloride). * Square box applies to adults only.
clarithromycin*	**Solid oral dosage form:** 500 mg. * For use in combination regimens for eradication of *H. Pylori* in adults.
doxycycline [a]	**Oral liquid:** 25 mg/5 ml [c]; 50 mg/5 ml (anhydrous) [c]. **Solid oral dosage form:** 50 mg [c]; 100 mg (as hyclate). [a] Use in children <8 years only for life-threatening infections when no alternative exists.
□ erythromycin	**Powder for injection:** 500 mg (as lactobionate) in vial. **Powder for oral liquid:** 125 mg/5 ml (as stearate **or** estolate **or** ethyl succinate). **Solid oral dosage form:** 250 mg (as stearate **or** estolate **or** ethyl succinate).

6. ANTI-INFECTIVE MEDICINES *(continued)*

□ gentamicin	**Injection:** 10 mg; 40 mg (as sulfate)/ml in 2-ml vial.
□ metronidazole	**Injection:** 500 mg in 100-ml vial. **Oral liquid:** 200 mg (as benzoate)/5 ml. **Suppository:** 500 mg; 1 g. **Tablet:** 200 mg to 500 mg.
nitrofurantoin	**Oral liquid:** 25 mg/5 ml [c]. **Tablet:** 100 mg.
spectinomycin	**Powder for injection:** 2 g (as hydrochloride) in vial.
sulfamethoxazole + trimethoprim	**Injection:** 80 mg + 16 mg/ml in 5-ml ampoule; 80 mg + 16 mg/ml in 10-ml ampoule. **Oral liquid:** 200 mg + 40 mg/5 ml. **Tablet:** 100 mg + 20 mg; 400 mg + 80 mg; 800 mg + 160 mg.
trimethoprim [a]	**Oral liquid:** 50 mg/5 ml [c]. **Tablet:** 100 mg; 200 mg. [a] >6 months.
Complementary List	
clindamycin	***Capsule:*** *150 mg (as hydrochloride).* ***Injection:*** *150 mg (as phosphate)/ml.* ***Oral liquid:*** *75 mg/5 ml (as palmitate)* [c].
vancomycin	***Powder for injection:*** *250 mg (as hydrochloride) in vial.*

6.2.3 *Antileprosy medicines*

Medicines used in the treatment of leprosy should never be used except in combination. Combination therapy is essential to prevent the emergence of drug resistance. Colour coded blister packs (MDT blister packs) containing standard two-medicine (paucibacillary leprosy) or three-medicine (multibacillary leprosy) combinations for adult and childhood leprosy should be used. MDT blister packs can be supplied free of charge through WHO.

clofazimine	**Capsule:** 50 mg; 100 mg.
dapsone	**Tablet:** 25 mg; 50 mg; 100 mg.
rifampicin	**Solid oral dosage form:** 150 mg; 300 mg.

6. ANTI-INFECTIVE MEDICINES *(continued)*

6.2.4 *Antituberculosis medicines*

ethambutol	**Oral liquid:** 25 mg/ml [c]. **Tablet:** 100 mg to 400 mg (hydrochloride).
ethambutol + isoniazid	**Tablet:** 400 mg + 150 mg.
ethambutol + isoniazid + pyrazinamide + rifampicin	**Tablet:** 275 mg + 75 mg + 400 mg + 150 mg.
ethambutol + isoniazid + rifampicin	**Tablet:** 275 mg + 75 mg + 150 mg.
isoniazid	**Oral liquid:** 50 mg/5 ml [c]. **Tablet:** 100 mg to 300 mg. **Tablet (scored):** 50 mg.
isoniazid + pyrazinamide + rifampicin	**Tablet:** 75 mg + 400 mg + 150 mg. 150 mg + 500 mg + 150 mg **(For intermittent use three times weekly).**
isoniazid + rifampicin	**Tablet:** 75 mg + 150 mg; 150 mg + 300 mg. 60 mg + 60 mg **(For intermittent use three times weekly).** 150 mg + 150 mg **(For intermittent use three times weekly).**
pyrazinamide	**Oral liquid:** 30 mg/ml [c]. **Tablet:** 400 mg. **Tablet (dispersible):** 150 mg. **Tablet (scored):** 150 mg.
rifabutin	**Capsule:** 150 mg.* * For use only in patients with HIV receiving protease inhibitors.
rifampicin	**Oral liquid:** 20 mg/ml [c]. **Solid oral dosage form:** 150 mg; 300 mg.
streptomycin	**Powder for injection:** 1 g (as sulfate) in vial.

6. ANTI-INFECTIVE MEDICINES *(continued)*

Complementary List

Reserve second-line drugs for the treatment of multidrug-resistant tuberculosis (MDR-TB) should be used in specialized centres adhering to WHO standards for TB control.

amikacin	***Powder for injection:*** *100 mg; 500 mg; 1 g (as sulfate) in vial.*
capreomycin	***Powder for injection:*** *1 g (as sulfate) in vial.*
cycloserine	***Solid oral dosage form:*** *250 mg.*
ethionamide	***Tablet:*** *125 mg; 250 mg.*
kanamycin	***Powder for injection:*** *1 g (as sulfate) in vial.*
*ofloxacin**	***Tablet:*** *200 mg; 400 mg.* * *Levofloxacin may be an alternative based on availability and programme considerations.*
p-aminosalicylic acid	***Granules:*** *4 g in sachet.* ***Tablet:*** *500 mg.*

6.3 Antifungal medicines

clotrimazole	**Vaginal cream:** 1%; 10%. **Vaginal tablet:** 100 mg; 500 mg.
□ fluconazole	**Capsule:** 50 mg. **Injection:** 2 mg/ml in vial. **Oral liquid:** 50 mg/5 ml.
griseofulvin	**Oral liquid:** 125 mg/5 ml [c]. **Solid oral dosage form:** 125 mg; 250 mg.
nystatin	**Lozenge:** 100 000 IU. **Oral liquid:** 50 mg/5 ml [c]; 100 000 IU/ml [c]. **Pessary:** 100 000 IU. **Tablet:** 100 000 IU; 500 000 IU.

Complementary List

amphotericin B	***Powder for injection:*** *50 mg in vial.* *As sodium deoxycholate* ***or*** *liposomal complex.*
flucytosine	***Capsule:*** *250 mg.* ***Infusion:*** *2.5 g in 250 ml.*
potassium iodide	***Saturated solution.***

6. ANTI-INFECTIVE MEDICINES *(continued)*

6.4 Antiviral medicines

6.4.1 *Antiherpes medicines*

□ aciclovir	**Oral liquid:** 200 mg/5 ml [c]. **Powder for injection:** 250 mg (as sodium salt) in vial. **Tablet:** 200 mg.

6.4.2 *Antiretrovirals*

Based on current evidence and experience of use, medicines in the following three classes of antiretrovirals are included as essential medicines for treatment and prevention of HIV (prevention of mother-to-child transmission and post-exposure prophylaxis). The Committee emphasizes the importance of using these products in accordance with global and national guidelines. The Committee recommends and endorses the use of fixed-dose combinations and the development of appropriate new fixed-dose combinations, including modified dosage forms, non-refrigerated products and paediatric dosage forms of assured pharmaceutical quality.

Scored tablets can be used in children and therefore can be considered for inclusion in the listing of tablets, provided adequate quality products are available.

6.4.2.1 *Nucleoside/Nucleotide reverse transcriptase inhibitors*

abacavir (ABC)	**Oral liquid:** 100 mg (as sulfate)/5 ml. **Tablet:** 300 mg (as sulfate).
didanosine (ddI)	**Buffered powder for oral liquid:** 100-mg; 167-mg; 250-mg packets. **Capsule (unbuffered enteric-coated):** 125 mg; 200 mg; 250 mg; 400 mg. **Tablet (buffered chewable, dispersible):** 25 mg; 50 mg; 100 mg; 150 mg; 200 mg.
emtricitabine (FTC)* [a]	**Capsule:** 200 mg. **Oral liquid:** 10 mg/ml. * FTC is an acceptable alternative to 3TC, based on knowledge of the pharmacology, the resistance patterns and clinical trials of antiretrovirals. [a] >3 months.
lamivudine (3TC)	**Oral liquid:** 50 mg/5 ml. **Tablet:** 150 mg.
stavudine (d4T)	**Capsule:** 15 mg; 20 mg; 30 mg. **Powder for oral liquid:** 5 mg/5 ml.

6. ANTI-INFECTIVE MEDICINES *(continued)*

tenofovir disoproxil fumarate (TDF)	**Tablet:** 300 mg (tenofovir disoproxil fumarate – equivalent to 245 mg tenofovir disoproxil).
zidovudine (ZDV **or** AZT)	**Capsule:** 100 mg; 250 mg. **Oral liquid:** 50 mg/5 ml. **Solution for IV infusion injection:** 10 mg/ml in 20-ml vial. **Tablet:** 300 mg.

6.4.2.2 *Non-nucleoside reverse transcriptase inhibitors*

efavirenz (EFV **or** EFZ) [a]	**Capsule:** 50 mg; 100 mg; 200 mg. **Oral liquid:** 150 mg/5 ml. **Tablet:** 600 mg. [a] >3 years **or** >10 kg weight.
nevirapine (NVP)	**Oral liquid:** 50 mg/5 ml. **Tablet:** 200 mg.

6.4.2.3 *Protease inhibitors*

Selection of protease inhibitor(s) from the Model List will need to be determined by each country after consideration of international and national treatment guidelines and experience. Ritonavir is recommended for use in combination as a pharmacological booster, and not as an antiretroviral in its own right. All other protease inhibitors should be used in boosted forms (e.g. with ritonavir).

atazanavir [a]	**Solid oral dosage form:** 100 mg; 150 mg; 300 mg (as sulfate). [a] >25 kg.
indinavir (IDV)	**Solid oral dosage form:** 400 mg (as sulfate).
lopinavir + ritonavir (LPV/r)	**Capsule:** 133.3 mg + 33.3 mg. **Oral liquid:** 400 mg + 100 mg/5 ml. **Tablet (heat stable):** 100 mg + 25 mg; 200 mg + 50 mg.
ritonavir	**Oral liquid:** 400 mg/5 ml. **Solid oral dosage form:** 100 mg. **Tablet (heat stable):** 25 mg; 100 mg.
saquinavir (SQV) [a]	**Solid oral dosage form:** 200 mg; 500 mg (as mesilate). [a] >25 kg.

6. ANTI-INFECTIVE MEDICINES *(continued)*

FIXED-DOSE COMBINATIONS

efavirenz + emtricitabine* + tenofovir	**Tablet:** 600 mg + 200 mg + 300 mg (disoproxil fumarate equivalent to 245 mg tenofovir disoproxil). * FTC is an acceptable alternative to 3TC, based on knowledge of the pharmacology, the resistance patterns and clinical trials of antiretrovirals.
emtricitabine* + tenofovir	**Tablet:** 200 mg + 300 mg (disoproxil fumarate equivalent to 245 mg tenofovir disoproxil). * FTC is an acceptable alternative to 3TC, based on knowledge of the pharmacology, the resistance patterns and clinical trials of antiretrovirals.
lamivudine + nevirapine + stavudine	**Tablet:** 150 mg + 200 mg + 30 mg. **Tablet (dispersible):** 30 mg + 50 mg + 6 mg [c]; 60 mg + 100 mg + 12 mg [c].
lamivudine + nevirapine + zidovudine	**Tablet:** 30 mg + 50 mg + 60 mg [c]; 150 mg + 200 mg + 300 mg.
lamivudine + zidovudine	**Tablet:** 30 mg + 60 mg [c]; 150 mg + 300 mg.

6.4.3 *Other antivirals*

oseltamivir*	**Capsule:** 30 mg; 45 mg; 75 mg (as phosphate). **Oral powder:** 12 mg/ml. * Oseltamivir should be used only in compliance with the WHO treatment guidelines, i.e. (1) for treatment of patients with severe or progressive clinical illness with confirmed or suspected influenza pandemic (H1N1) 2009, (2) for the treatment of patients with confirmed or suspected but uncomplicated illness due to pandemic influenza virus infection who were in higher risk groups, most notably for pregnant women and children under 2 years of age.
ribavirin*	**Injection for intravenous administration:** 800 mg and 1 g in 10-ml phosphate buffer solution. **Solid oral dosage form:** 200 mg; 400 mg; 600 mg. * For the treatment of viral haemorrhagic fevers only.

6.5 Antiprotozoal medicines

6.5.1 *Antiamoebic and antigiardiasis medicines*

diloxanide [a]	**Tablet:** 500 mg (furoate). [a] >25 kg.

6. ANTI-INFECTIVE MEDICINES *(continued)*

□ metronidazole	**Injection:** 500 mg in 100-ml vial. **Oral liquid:** 200 mg (as benzoate)/5 ml. **Tablet:** 200 mg to 500 mg.

6.5.2 *Antileishmaniasis medicines*

amphotericin B	**Powder for injection:** 50 mg in vial. As sodium deoxycholate **or** liposomal complex.
miltefosine	**Solid oral dosage form:** 10 mg; 50 mg.
paromomycin	**Solution for intramuscular injection:** 750 mg of paromomycin base (as the sulfate).
sodium stibogluconate **or** meglumine antimoniate	**Injection:** 100 mg/ml, 1 vial = 30 ml **or** 30%, equivalent to approximately 8.1% antimony (pentavalent) in 5-ml ampoule.

6.5.3 *Antimalarial medicines*

6.5.3.1 *For curative treatment*

Medicines for the treatment of *P. falciparum* malaria cases should be used in combination. The list currently recommends combinations according to treatment guidelines. The Committee recognizes that not all of these FDCs exist and encourages their development and rigorous testing. The Committee also encourages development and testing of rectal dosage formulations.

amodiaquine*	**Tablet:** 153 mg **or** 200 mg (as hydrochloride). * To be used in combination with artesunate 50 mg.
artemether*	**Oily injection:** 80 mg/ml in 1-ml ampoule. * For use in the management of severe malaria.
artemether + lumefantrine*	**Tablet:** 20 mg + 120 mg. **Tablet (dispersible):** 20 mg + 120 mg [c]. * Not recommended in the first trimester of pregnancy **or** in children below 5 kg.
artesunate*	**Injection:** ampoules, containing 60 mg anhydrous artesunic acid with a separate ampoule of 5% sodium bicarbonate solution. For use in the management of severe malaria. **Rectal dosage form:** 50 mg [c]; 200 mg capsules (for pre-referral treatment of severe malaria only; patients should be taken to an appropriate health facility for follow-up care) [c]. **Tablet:** 50 mg. * To be used in combination with either amodiaquine, mefloquine **or** sulfadoxine + pyrimethamine.

6. ANTI-INFECTIVE MEDICINES *(continued)*

artesunate + amodiaquine*	**Tablet:** 25 mg + 67.5 mg; 50 mg + 135 mg; 100 mg + 270 mg. * Other combinations that deliver the target doses required such as 153 mg **or** 200 mg (as hydrochloride) with 50 mg artesunate can be alternatives.
chloroquine*	**Oral liquid:** 50 mg (as phosphate **or** sulfate)/5 ml. **Tablet:** 100 mg; 150 mg (as phosphate **or** sulfate). * For use only for the treatment of *P. vivax* infection.
doxycycline*	**Capsule:** 100 mg (as hydrochloride **or** hyclate). **Tablet (dispersible):** 100 mg (as monohydrate). * For use only in combination with quinine.
mefloquine*	**Tablet:** 250 mg (as hydrochloride). * To be used in combination with artesunate 50 mg.
primaquine*	**Tablet:** 7.5 mg; 15 mg (as diphosphate). * Only for use to achieve radical cure of *P. vivax* and *P. ovale* infections, given for 14 days.
quinine*	**Injection:** 300 mg quinine hydrochloride/ml in 2-ml ampoule. **Tablet:** 300 mg (quinine sulfate) **or** 300 mg (quinine bisulfate). * For use only in the management of severe malaria, and should be used in combination with doxycycline.
sulfadoxine + pyrimethamine*	**Tablet:** 500 mg + 25 mg. * Only in combination with artesunate 50 mg.

6.5.3.2 *For prophylaxis*

chloroquine*	**Oral liquid:** 50 mg (as phosphate **or** sulfate)/5 ml. **Tablet:** 150 mg (as phosphate **or** sulfate). * For use only in central American regions, for use for *P. vivax*.
doxycycline [a]	**Solid oral dosage form:** 100 mg (as hydrochloride **or** hyclate). [a] >8 years.
mefloquine [a]	**Tablet:** 250 mg (as hydrochloride). [a] >5 kg **or** >3 months.
proguanil*	**Tablet:** 100 mg (as hydrochloride). * For use only in combination with chloroquine.

6. ANTI-INFECTIVE MEDICINES *(continued)*

6.5.4 *Antipneumocystosis and antitoxoplasmosis medicines*

pyrimethamine	**Tablet:** 25 mg.
sulfadiazine	**Tablet:** 500 mg.
sulfamethoxazole + trimethoprim	**Injection:** 80 mg + 16 mg/ml in 5-ml ampoule; 80 mg + 16 mg/ml in 10-ml ampoule. **Oral liquid:** 200 mg + 40 mg/5 ml [c]. **Tablet:** 100 mg + 20 mg; 400 mg + 80 mg [c].
Complementary List	
pentamidine	***Tablet:*** *200 mg; 300 mg (as isethionate).*

6.5.5 *Antitrypanosomal medicines*

6.5.5.1 *African trypanosomiasis*

Medicines for the treatment of 1st stage African trypanosomiasis

pentamidine*	**Powder for injection:** 200 mg (as isetionate) in vial. * To be used for the treatment of *Trypanosoma brucei gambiense* infection.
suramin sodium*	**Powder for injection:** 1 g in vial. * To be used for the treatment of the initial phase of *Trypanosoma brucei rhodesiense* infection.

Medicines for the treatment of 2nd stage African trypanosomiasis

eflornithine*	**Injection:** 200 mg (hydrochloride)/ml in 100-ml bottle. * To be used for the treatment of *Trypanosoma brucei gambiense* infection.
melarsoprol	**Injection:** 3.6% solution, 5-ml ampoule (180 mg of active compound).
nifurtimox*	**Tablet:** 120 mg. * Only to be used in combination with eflornithine, for the treatment of *Trypanosoma brucei gambiense* infection.
Complementary List [c]	
melarsoprol	***Injection:*** *3.6% solution in 5-ml ampoule (180 mg of active compound).*

6. ANTI-INFECTIVE MEDICINES *(continued)*

6.5.5.2 *American trypanosomiasis*

benznidazole	**Tablet:** 100 mg.
nifurtimox	**Tablet:** 30 mg; 120 mg; 250 mg.

7. ANTIMIGRAINE MEDICINES

7.1 For treatment of acute attack

acetylsalicylic acid	**Tablet:** 300 mg to 500 mg.
ibuprofen [c]	**Tablet:** 200 mg; 400 mg.
paracetamol	**Oral liquid:** 125 mg/5 ml [c]. **Tablet:** 300 mg to 500 mg.

7.2 For prophylaxis

□ propranolol	**Tablet:** 20 mg; 40 mg (hydrochloride).

8. ANTINEOPLASTIC, IMMUNOSUPPRESSIVES AND MEDICINES USED IN PALLIATIVE CARE

8.1 Immunosuppressive medicines

Complementary List

azathioprine	***Powder for injection:*** *100 mg (as sodium salt) in vial.* ***Tablet (scored):*** *50 mg.*
ciclosporin	***Capsule:*** *25 mg.* ***Concentrate for injection:*** *50 mg/ml in 1-ml ampoule for organ transplantation.*

8.2 Cytotoxic and adjuvant medicines

Complementary List

allopurinol [c]	***Tablet:*** *100 mg; 300 mg.*
asparaginase	***Powder for injection:*** *10 000 IU in vial.*
bleomycin	***Powder for injection:*** *15 mg (as sulfate) in vial.*
calcium folinate	***Injection:*** *3 mg/ml in 10-ml ampoule.* ***Tablet:*** *15 mg.*
□ *carboplatin*	***Injection:*** *50 mg/5 ml; 150 mg/15 ml; 450 mg/45 ml; 600 mg/60 ml.*
chlorambucil	***Tablet:*** *2 mg.*

8. ANTINEOPLASTIC, IMMUNOSUPPRESSIVES AND MEDICINES USED IN PALLIATIVE CARE *(continued)*

cyclophosphamide	***Powder for injection:*** *500 mg in vial.* ***Tablet:*** *25 mg.*
cytarabine	***Powder for injection:*** *100 mg in vial.*
dacarbazine	***Powder for injection:*** *100 mg in vial.*
dactinomycin	***Powder for injection:*** *500 micrograms in vial.*
daunorubicin	***Powder for injection:*** *50 mg (hydrochloride) in vial.*
docetaxel	***Injection:*** *20 mg/ml; 40 mg/ml.*
doxorubicin	***Powder for injection:*** *10 mg; 50 mg (hydrochloride) in vial.*
etoposide	***Capsule:*** *100 mg.* ***Injection:*** *20 mg/ml in 5-ml ampoule.*
fluorouracil	***Injection:*** *50 mg/ml in 5-ml ampoule.*
hydroxycarbamide	***Solid oral dosage form:*** *200 mg; 250 mg; 300 mg; 400 mg; 500 mg; 1 g.*
ifosfamide	***Powder for injection:*** *1 g vial; 2 g vial.*
mercaptopurine	***Tablet:*** *50 mg.*
mesna	***Injection:*** *100 mg/ml in 4-ml and 10-ml ampoules.* ***Tablet:*** *400 mg; 600 mg.*
methotrexate	***Powder for injection:*** *50 mg (as sodium salt) in vial.* ***Tablet:*** *2.5 mg (as sodium salt).*
paclitaxel	***Powder for injection:*** *6 mg/ml.*
procarbazine	***Capsule:*** *50 mg (as hydrochloride).*
thioguanine [c]	***Solid oral dosage form:*** *40 mg.*
vinblastine	***Powder for injection:*** *10 mg (sulfate) in vial.*
vincristine	***Powder for injection:*** *1 mg; 5 mg (sulfate) in vial.*

8.3 Hormones and antihormones

Complementary List

dexamethasone	***Injection:*** *4 mg/ml in 1-ml ampoule (as disodium phosphate salt).* ***Oral liquid:*** *2 mg/5 ml* [c].

8. ANTINEOPLASTIC, IMMUNOSUPPRESSIVES AND MEDICINES USED IN PALLIATIVE CARE *(continued)*

hydrocortisone	***Powder for injection:*** *100 mg (as sodium succinate) in vial.*
methylprednisolone [c]	***Injection:*** *40 mg/ml (as sodium succinate) in 1-ml single dose vial and 5-ml multidose vials; 80 mg/ml (as sodium succinate) in 1-ml single dose vial.*
□ *prednisolone*	***Oral liquid:*** *5 mg/ml* [c]. ***Tablet:*** *5 mg; 25 mg.*
tamoxifen	***Tablet:*** *10 mg; 20 mg (as citrate).*

8.4 Medicines used in palliative care

The WHO Expert Committee recognizes the importance of listing specific medicines in the Palliative Care Section. Some medicines currently used in palliative care are included in the relevant sections of the Model List, according to their therapeutic use, e.g. analgesics. The Guidelines for Palliative Care that were referenced in the previous list are in need of update. The Committee expects applications for medicines needed for palliative care to be submitted for the next meeting.

amitriptyline [c]	**Tablet:** 10 mg; 25 mg.
cyclizine [c]	**Injection:** 50 mg/ml. **Tablet:** 50 mg.
dexamethasone [c]	**Injection:** 4 mg/ml in 1-ml ampoule (as disodium phosphate salt). **Tablet:** 2 mg.
diazepam [c]	**Injection:** 5 mg/ml. **Oral liquid:** 2 mg/5 ml. **Rectal solution:** 2.5 mg; 5 mg; 10 mg. **Tablet:** 5 mg; 10 mg.
docusate sodium [c]	**Capsule:** 100 mg. **Oral liquid:** 50 mg/5 ml.
fluoxetine [a] [c]	**Solid oral dosage form:** 20 mg (as hydrochloride). [a] >8 years.
hyoscine hydrobromide [c]	**Injection:** 400 micrograms/ml; 600 micrograms/ml. **Transdermal patches:** 1 mg/72 hours.

8. ANTINEOPLASTIC, IMMUNOSUPPRESSIVES AND MEDICINES USED IN PALLIATIVE CARE *(continued)*

ibuprofen [a] [c]	**Oral liquid:** 200 mg/5 ml. **Tablet:** 200 mg; 400 mg; 600 mg. [a] Not in children less than 3 months.
lactulose [c]	**Oral liquid:** 3.1–3.7 g/5 ml.
midazolam [c]	**Injection:** 1 mg/ml; 5 mg/ml.
morphine [c]	**Granules (modified release) (to mix with water):** 20 mg; 30 mg; 60 mg; 100 mg; 200 mg. **Injection:** 10 mg/ml. **Oral liquid:** 10 mg/5 ml. **Tablet (controlled release):** 10 mg; 30 mg; 60 mg. **Tablet (immediate release):** 10 mg.
ondansetron [c] [a]	**Injection:** 2 mg base/ml in 2-ml ampoule (as hydrochloride). **Oral liquid:** 4 mg base/5 ml. **Solid oral dosage form:** Eq 4 mg base; Eq 8 mg base. [a] >1 month.
senna [c]	**Oral liquid:** 7.5 mg/5 ml.

9. ANTIPARKINSONISM MEDICINES

biperiden	**Injection:** 5 mg (lactate) in 1-ml ampoule. **Tablet:** 2 mg (hydrochloride).
levodopa + □ carbidopa	**Tablet:** 100 mg + 10 mg; 250 mg + 25 mg.

10. MEDICINES AFFECTING THE BLOOD

10.1 Antianaemia medicines

ferrous salt	**Oral liquid:** equivalent to 25 mg iron (as sulfate)/ml. **Tablet:** equivalent to 60 mg iron.
ferrous salt + folic acid	**Tablet:** equivalent to 60 mg iron + 400 micrograms folic acid (Nutritional supplement for use during pregnancy).
folic acid	**Tablet:** 1 mg; 5 mg.
hydroxocobalamin	**Injection:** 1 mg (as acetate, hydrochloride **or** as sulfate) in 1-ml ampoule.

10. MEDICINES AFFECTING THE BLOOD *(continued)*

10.2 Medicines affecting coagulation

heparin sodium	**Injection:** 1000 IU/ml; 5000 IU/ml; 20 000 IU/ml in 1-ml ampoule.
phytomenadione	**Injection:** 1 mg/ml [c]; 10 mg/ml in 5-ml ampoule. **Tablet:** 10 mg.
protamine sulfate	**Injection:** 10 mg/ml in 5-ml ampoule.
tranexamic acid	**Injection:** 100 mg/ml in 10-ml ampoule.
□ warfarin	**Tablet:** 1 mg; 2 mg; 5 mg (sodium salt).
***Complementary List* [c]**	
heparin sodium	***Injection:** 1000 IU/ml; 5000 IU/ml in 1-ml ampoule.*
protamine sulfate	***Injection:** 10 mg/ml in 5-ml ampoule.*
□ *warfarin*	***Tablet:** 0.5 mg; 1 mg; 2 mg; 5 mg (sodium salt).*

10.3 Other medicines for haemoglobinopathies

Complementary List	
*deferoxamine**	***Powder for injection:** 500 mg (mesilate) in vial.* * *Deferasirox oral form may be an alternative, depending on cost and availability.*
hydroxycarbamide	***Solid oral dosage form:** 200 mg; 500 mg; 1 g.*

11. BLOOD PRODUCTS AND PLASMA SUBSTITUTES

11.1 Plasma substitutes

□ dextran 70*	**Injectable solution:** 6%. * Polygeline, injectable solution, 3.5% is considered as equivalent.

11.2 Plasma fractions for specific use

All plasma fractions should comply with the WHO Requirements for the Collection, Processing and Quality Control of Blood, Blood Components and Plasma Derivatives (Revised 1992). (WHO Technical Report Series, No. 840, 1994, Annex 2).

Complementary List	
□ *factor VIII concentrate*	***Dried.***
□ *factor IX complex (coagulation factors, II, VII, IX, X) concentrate*	***Dried.***

11. BLOOD PRODUCTS AND PLASMA SUBSTITUTES *(continued)*

human normal immunoglobulin	***Intramuscular administration:*** *16% protein solution.** ***Intravenous administration:*** *5%; 10% protein solution.*** ***Subcutaneous administration:*** *15%; 16% protein solution.** ** Indicated for primary immune deficiency.* *** Indicated for primary immune deficiency and Kawasaki disease.*

12. CARDIOVASCULAR MEDICINES

12.1 Antianginal medicines

□ bisoprolol*	**Tablet:** 1.25 mg; 5 mg. * □ includes metoprolol and carvedilol as alternatives.
glyceryl trinitrate	**Tablet (sublingual):** 500 micrograms.
□ isosorbide dinitrate	**Tablet (sublingual):** 5 mg.
verapamil	**Tablet:** 40 mg; 80 mg (hydrochloride).

12.2 Antiarrhythmic medicines

□ bisoprolol*	**Tablet:** 1.25 mg; 5 mg. * □ includes metoprolol and carvedilol as alternatives.
digoxin	**Injection:** 250 micrograms/ml in 2-ml ampoule. **Oral liquid:** 50 micrograms/ml. **Tablet:** 62.5 micrograms; 250 micrograms.
epinephrine (adrenaline)	**Injection:** 100 micrograms/ml (as acid tartrate **or** hydrochloride) in 10-ml ampoule.
lidocaine	**Injection:** 20 mg (hydrochloride)/ml in 5-ml ampoule.
verapamil	**Injection:** 2.5 mg (hydrochloride)/ml in 2-ml ampoule. **Tablet:** 40 mg; 80 mg (hydrochloride).
Complementary List	
amiodarone	***Injection:*** *50 mg/ml in 3-ml ampoule (hydrochloride).* ***Tablet (HCl):*** *100 mg; 200 mg; 400 mg (hydrochloride).*

12. CARDIOVASCULAR MEDICINES *(continued)*

12.3 Antihypertensive medicines

□ amlodipine	**Tablet:** 5 mg (as maleate, mesylate **or** besylate).
□ bisoprolol*	**Tablet:** 1.25 mg; 5 mg. * □ includes metoprolol and carvedilol as alternatives.
□ enalapril	**Tablet:** 2.5 mg; 5 mg (as hydrogen maleate).
hydralazine*	**Powder for injection:** 20 mg (hydrochloride) in ampoule. **Tablet:** 25 mg; 50 mg (hydrochloride). * Hydralazine is listed for use in the acute management of severe pregnancy-induced hypertension only. Its use in the treatment of essential hypertension is not recommended in view of the availability of more evidence of efficacy and safety of other medicines.
□ hydrochlorothiazide	**Oral liquid:** 50 mg/5 ml. **Solid oral dosage form:** 12.5 mg; 25 mg.
methyldopa*	**Tablet:** 250 mg. * Methyldopa is listed for use in the management of pregnancy-induced hypertension only. Its use in the treatment of essential hypertension is not recommended in view of the availability of more evidence of efficacy and safety of other medicines.
Complementary List	
sodium nitroprusside	***Powder for infusion:** 50 mg in ampoule.*

12.4 Medicines used in heart failure

□ bisoprolol*	**Tablet:** 1.25 mg; 5 mg. * □ includes metoprolol and carvedilol as alternatives.
digoxin	**Injection:** 250 micrograms/ml in 2-ml ampoule. **Oral liquid:** 50 micrograms/ml. **Tablet:** 62.5 micrograms; 250 micrograms.
□ enalapril	**Tablet:** 2.5 mg; 5 mg (as hydrogen maleate).
□ furosemide	**Injection:** 10 mg/ml in 2-ml ampoule. **Oral liquid:** 20 mg/5 ml [c]. **Tablet:** 40 mg.
□ hydrochlorothiazide	**Oral liquid:** 50 mg/5 ml. **Solid oral dosage form:** 25 mg.

12. CARDIOVASCULAR MEDICINES *(continued)*

Complementary List

dopamine	***Injection:*** *40 mg/ml (hydrochloride) in 5-ml vial.*

12.5 Antithrombotic medicines

acetylsalicylic acid	**Tablet:** 100 mg.

Complementary List

streptokinase	***Powder for injection:*** *1.5 million IU in vial.*

12.6 Lipid-lowering agents

□ simvastatin*	**Tablet:** 5 mg; 10 mg; 20 mg; 40 mg. * For use in high-risk patients.

13. DERMATOLOGICAL MEDICINES (topical)

13.1 Antifungal medicines

□ miconazole	**Cream or ointment:** 2% (nitrate).
selenium sulfide	**Detergent-based suspension:** 2%.
sodium thiosulfate	**Solution:** 15%.
terbinafine	**Cream:** 1% **or Ointment:** 1% terbinafine hydrochloride.

13.2 Anti-infective medicines

mupirocin	**Cream (as mupirocin calcium):** 2%. **Ointment:** 2%.
potassium permanganate	**Aqueous solution:** 1:10 000.
silver sulfadiazine [a]	**Cream:** 1%. [a] >2 months.

13.3 Anti-inflammatory and antipruritic medicines

□ betamethasone [a]	**Cream or ointment:** 0.1% (as valerate). [a] Hydrocortisone preferred in neonates.
□ calamine	**Lotion.**
□ hydrocortisone	**Cream or ointment:** 1% (acetate).

13. DERMATOLOGICAL MEDICINES (topical) *(continued)*

13.4 Medicines affecting skin differentiation and proliferation

benzoyl peroxide	**Cream or lotion:** 5%.
coal tar	**Solution:** 5%.
dithranol*	**Ointment:** 0.1% to 2%. * The Expert Committee has requested a review of the comparative effectiveness and safety, for possible deletion of this medicine at its next meeting.
fluorouracil	**Ointment:** 5%.
□ podophyllum resin	**Solution:** 10% to 25%.
salicylic acid	**Solution:** 5%.
urea	**Cream or ointment:** 5%; 10%.

13.5 Scabicides and pediculicides

□ benzyl benzoate [a]	**Lotion:** 25%. [a] >2 years.
permethrin	**Cream:** 5%. **Lotion:** 1%.

14. DIAGNOSTIC AGENTS

14.1 Ophthalmic medicines

fluorescein	**Eye drops:** 1% (sodium salt).
□ tropicamide	**Eye drops:** 0.5%.

14.2 Radiocontrast media

□ amidotrizoate	**Injection:** 140 mg to 420 mg iodine (as sodium **or** meglumine salt)/ml in 20-ml ampoule.
barium sulfate	**Aqueous suspension.**
□ iohexol	**Injection:** 140 mg to 350 mg iodine/ml in 5-ml; 10-ml; 20-ml ampoules.
Complementary List	
barium sulfate [c]	***Aqueous suspension.***
□ *meglumine iotroxate*	***Solution:*** *5 g to 8 g iodine in 100 ml to 250 ml.*

15. DISINFECTANTS AND ANTISEPTICS

15.1 Antiseptics

☐ chlorhexidine	**Solution:** 5% (digluconate); 20% (digluconate) (needs to be diluted prior to use for cord care) [c].
☐ ethanol	**Solution:** 70% (denatured).
☐ polyvidone iodine	**Solution:** 10% (equivalent to 1% available iodine).

15.2 Disinfectants

☐ chlorine base compound	**Powder:** (0.1% available chlorine) for solution.
☐ chloroxylenol	**Solution:** 4.8%.
glutaral	**Solution:** 2%.

16. DIURETICS

amiloride	**Tablet:** 5 mg (hydrochloride).
☐ furosemide	**Injection:** 10 mg/ml in 2-ml ampoule. **Oral liquid:** 20 mg/5 ml [c]. **Tablet:** 10 mg [c]; 20 mg [c]; 40 mg.
☐ hydrochlorothiazide	**Solid oral dosage form:** 25 mg.
mannitol	**Injectable solution:** 10%; 20%.
spironolactone	**Tablet:** 25 mg.
***Complementary List* [c]**	
☐ *hydrochlorothiazide*	***Tablet (scored):*** *25 mg.*
mannitol	***Injectable solution:*** *10%; 20%.*
spironolactone	***Oral liquid:*** *5 mg/5 ml; 10 mg/5 ml; 25 mg/5 ml.* ***Tablet:*** *25 mg.*

17. GASTROINTESTINAL MEDICINES

***Complementary List* [c]**	
☐ *pancreatic enzymes*	*Age-appropriate formulations and doses including lipase, protease and amylase.*

17.1 Antiulcer medicines

☐ omeprazole	**Powder for oral liquid:** 20 mg; 40 mg sachets. **Solid oral dosage form:** 10 mg; 20 mg; 40 mg.

17. GASTROINTESTINAL MEDICINES *(continued)*	
□ ranitidine*	**Injection:** 25 mg/ml (as hydrochloride) in 2-ml ampoule. **Oral liquid:** 75 mg/5 ml (as hydrochloride). **Tablet:** 150 mg (as hydrochloride). * The Expert Committee has requested a review of the comparative effectiveness and safety, for possible deletion of this class of medicine at its next meeting.
17.2 Antiemetic medicines	
dexamethasone	**Injection:** 4 mg/ml in 1-ml ampoule (as disodium phosphate salt). **Oral liquid:** 0.5 mg/5 ml; 2 mg/5 ml. **Solid oral dosage form:** 0.5 mg; 0.75 mg; 1.5 mg; 4 mg.
metoclopramide [a]	**Injection:** 5 mg (hydrochloride)/ml in 2-ml ampoule. **Oral liquid:** 5 mg/5 ml [c]. **Tablet:** 10 mg (hydrochloride). [a] Not in neonates.
ondansetron [a]	**Injection:** 2 mg base/ml in 2-ml ampoule (as hydrochloride). **Oral liquid:** 4 mg base/5 ml. **Solid oral dosage form:** Eq 4 mg base; Eq 8 mg base; Eq 24 mg base. [a] >1 month.
17.3 Anti-inflammatory medicines	
□ sulfasalazine	**Retention enema.** **Suppository:** 500 mg. **Tablet:** 500 mg.
Complementary List	
□ hydrocortisone	***Retention enema.*** ***Suppository:** 25 mg (acetate).* (the □ only applies to hydrocortisone retention enema).
17.4 Laxatives	
□ senna	**Tablet:** 7.5 mg (sennosides) (or traditional dosage forms).

17. GASTROINTESTINAL MEDICINES *(continued)*

17.5 Medicines used in diarrhoea

17.5.1 *Oral rehydration*

oral rehydration salts	glucose:	75 mEq
	sodium:	75 mEq **or** mmol/L
	chloride:	65 mEq **or** mmol/L
	potassium:	20 mEq **or** mmol/L
	citrate:	10 mmol/L
	osmolarity:	245 mOsm/L
	glucose:	13.5 g/L
	sodium chloride:	2.6 g/L
	potassium chloride:	1.5 g/L
	trisodium citrate dihydrate+:	2.9 g/L

+ trisodium citrate dihydrate may be replaced by sodium hydrogen carbonate (sodium bicarbonate) 2.5 g/L. However, as the stability of this latter formulation is very poor under tropical conditions, it is only recommended when manufactured for immediate use.

Powder for dilution in 200 ml; 500 ml; 1 L.

17.5.2 *Medicines for diarrhoea in children*

zinc sulfate* — **Solid oral dosage form:** 20 mg.

* In acute diarrhoea zinc sulfate should be used as an adjunct to oral rehydration salts.

18. HORMONES, OTHER ENDOCRINE MEDICINES AND CONTRACEPTIVES

18.1 Adrenal hormones and synthetic substitutes

fludrocortisone	**Tablet:** 100 micrograms (acetate).
hydrocortisone	**Tablet:** 5 mg; 10 mg; 20 mg.

18.2 Androgens

Complementary List

testosterone	***Injection:** 200 mg (enanthate) in 1-ml ampoule.*

18.3 Contraceptives

18.3.1 *Oral hormonal contraceptives*

☐ ethinylestradiol + ☐ levonorgestrel	**Tablet:** 30 micrograms + 150 micrograms.

ONES, OTHER ENDOCRINE MEDICINES AND CONTRACEPTIVES *(continued)*

□ e... estradiol + □ norethisterone	**Tablet:** 35 micrograms + 1 mg.
levonorgestrel	**Tablet:** 30 micrograms; 750 micrograms (pack of two); 1.5 mg.

18.3.2 ***Injectable hormonal contraceptives***

estradiol cypionate + medroxyprogesterone acetate	**Injection:** 5 mg + 25 mg.
medroxyprogesterone acetate	**Depot injection:** 150 mg/ml in 1-ml vial.
norethisterone enantate	**Oily solution:** 200 mg/ml in 1-ml ampoule.

18.3.3 ***Intrauterine devices***

copper-containing device

18.3.4 ***Barrier methods***

condoms

diaphragms

18.3.5 ***Implantable contraceptives***

levonorgestrel-releasing implant	Two-rod levonorgestrel-releasing implant, each rod containing 75 mg of levonorgestrel (150 mg total).

18.4 Estrogens

18.5 Insulins and other medicines used for diabetes

glibenclamide	**Tablet:** 2.5 mg; 5 mg.
glucagon	**Injection:** 1 mg/ml.
insulin injection (soluble)	**Injection:** 40 IU/ml in 10-ml vial; 100 IU/ml in 10-ml vial.
intermediate-acting insulin	**Injection:** 40 IU/ml in 10-ml vial; 100 IU/ml in 10-ml vial (as compound insulin zinc suspension **or** isophane insulin).
metformin	**Tablet:** 500 mg (hydrochloride).
Complementary List **[c]**	
metformin	***Tablet:*** *500 mg (hydrochloride).*

18. HORMONES, OTHER ENDOCRINE MEDICINES AND CONTRACEPTIVES *(continued)*

18.6 Ovulation inducers

Complementary List

clomifene	***Tablet:*** *50 mg (citrate).*

18.7 Progestogens

□ medroxyprogesterone acetate	**Tablet:** 5 mg.

18.8 Thyroid hormones and antithyroid medicines

levothyroxine	**Tablet:** 25 micrograms [c]; 50 micrograms; 100 micrograms (sodium salt).
potassium iodide	**Tablet:** 60 mg.
□ propylthiouracil	**Tablet:** 50 mg.

Complementary List [c]

Lugol's solution	***Oral liquid:*** *about 130 mg total iodine/ml.*
potassium iodide	***Tablet:*** *60 mg.*
propylthiouracil	***Tablet:*** *50 mg.*

19. IMMUNOLOGICALS

19.1 Diagnostic agents

All tuberculins should comply with the WHO Requirements for Tuberculins (Revised 1985). WHO Expert Committee on Biological Standardization. Thirty-sixth report. (*WHO Technical Report Series*, No. 745, 1987, Annex 1).

tuberculin, purified protein derivative (PPD)	**Injection.**

19.2 Sera and immunoglobulins

All plasma fractions should comply with the WHO Requirements for the Collection, Processing and Quality Control of Blood, Blood Components and Plasma Derivatives (Revised 1992). WHO Expert Committee on Biological Standardization. Forty-third report. (*WHO Technical Report Series*, No. 840, 1994, Annex 2).

anti-D immunoglobulin (human)	**Injection:** 250 micrograms in single-dose vial.
antitetanus immunoglobulin (human)	**Injection:** 500 IU in vial.
antivenom immunoglobulin*	**Injection.** * Exact type to be defined locally.

19. IMMUNOLOGICALS *(continued)*	
diphtheria antitoxin	**Injection:** 10 000 IU; 20 000 IU in vial.
□ rabies immunoglobulin	**Injection:** 150 IU/ml in vial.

19.3 Vaccines

Selection of vaccines from the Model List will need to be determined by each country after consideration of international recommendations, epidemiology and national priorities. The list below details the vaccines for which there is either a recommendation from the Strategic Advisory Group of Experts on Immunization (SAGE) (http://www.who.int/immunization/sage_conclusions/en/index.html) and/or a WHO position paper (http://www.who.int/immunization/documents/positionpapers/en/index.html). This site will be updated as new position papers are published and contains the most recent information and recommendations.

All vaccines should comply with the WHO Requirements for Biological Substances.

BCG vaccine

cholera vaccine

diphtheria vaccine

Haemophilus influenzae type b vaccine

hepatitis A vaccine

hepatitis B vaccine

influenza vaccine

Japanese encephalitis vaccine

measles vaccine

meningococcal meningitis vaccine

mumps vaccine

pertussis vaccine

pneumococcal vaccine

poliomyelitis vaccine

rabies vaccine

rotavirus vaccine

rubella vaccine

tetanus vaccine

typhoid vaccine

19. IMMUNOLOGICALS *(continued)*

varicella vaccine

yellow fever vaccine

20. MUSCLE RELAXANTS (PERIPHERALLY-ACTING) AND CHOLINESTERASE INHIBITORS

The Expert Committee has requested a review of this section at its next meeting.

Medicine	Dosage form and strength
□ atracurium	**Injection:** 10 mg/ml (besylate).
neostigmine	**Injection:** 500 micrograms in 1-ml ampoule; 2.5 mg (metilsulfate) in 1-ml ampoule. **Tablet:** 15 mg (bromide).
suxamethonium	**Injection:** 50 mg (chloride)/ml in 2-ml ampoule. **Powder for injection** (chloride), in vial.
□ vecuronium [c]	**Powder for injection:** 10 mg (bromide) in vial.
Complementary List	
pyridostigmine	***Injection:** 1 mg in 1-ml ampoule.* ***Tablet:** 60 mg (bromide).*
□ *vecuronium*	***Powder for injection:** 10 mg (bromide) in vial.*

21. OPHTHALMOLOGICAL PREPARATIONS

This section will be reviewed at the next meeting of the Expert Committee.

21.1 Anti-infective agents

Medicine	Dosage form and strength
aciclovir	**Ointment:** 3% W/W.
□ gentamicin	**Solution (eye drops):** 0.3% (sulfate).
□ tetracycline	**Eye ointment:** 1% (hydrochloride).

21.2 Anti-inflammatory agents

Medicine	Dosage form and strength
□ prednisolone	**Solution (eye drops):** 0.5% (sodium phosphate).

21.3 Local anaesthetics

Medicine	Dosage form and strength
□ tetracaine [a]	**Solution (eye drops):** 0.5% (hydrochloride). [a] Not in preterm neonates.

21.4 Miotics and antiglaucoma medicines

Medicine	Dosage form and strength
acetazolamide	**Tablet:** 250 mg.

21. OPHTHALMOLOGICAL PREPARATIONS *(continued)*

□ pilocarpine	**Solution (eye drops):** 2%; 4% (hydrochloride **or** nitrate).
□ timolol	**Solution (eye drops):** 0.25%; 0.5% (as hydrogen maleate).

21.5 Mydriatics

atropine* [a]	**Solution (eye drops):** 0.1%; 0.5%; 1% (sulfate). * [c] **Or** homatropine (hydrobromide) **or** cyclopentolate (hydrochloride). [a] >3 months.

Complementary List

epinephrine (adrenaline)	***Solution (eye drops):*** *2% (as hydrochloride).*

22. OXYTOCICS AND ANTIOXYTOCICS

22.1 Oxytocics

□ ergometrine	**Injection:** 200 micrograms (hydrogen maleate) in 1-ml ampoule.
misoprostol	**Tablet:** 200 micrograms.* * For management of incomplete abortion and miscarriage, and for prevention of postpartum haemorrhage where oxytocin is not available or cannot be safely used. **Vaginal tablet:** 25 micrograms.* * Only for use for induction of labour where appropriate facilities are available.
oxytocin	**Injection:** 10 IU in 1 ml.

Complementary List

mifepristone – misoprostol** *Where permitted under national law and where culturally acceptable.*	***Tablet*** *200 mg –* ***tablet*** *200 micrograms.* * *Requires close medical supervision.*

22.2 Antioxytocics (tocolytics)

nifedipine	**Immediate-release capsule:** 10 mg.

23. PERITONEAL DIALYSIS SOLUTION

Complementary List

intraperitoneal dialysis solution (of appropriate composition)	***Parenteral solution.***

24. MEDICINES FOR MENTAL AND BEHAVIOURAL DISORDERS

24.1 Medicines used in psychotic disorders

□ chlorpromazine	**Injection:** 25 mg (hydrochloride)/ml in 2-ml ampoule. **Oral liquid:** 25 mg (hydrochloride)/5 ml. **Tablet:** 100 mg (hydrochloride).
□ fluphenazine	**Injection:** 25 mg (decanoate **or** enantate) in 1-ml ampoule.
□ haloperidol	**Injection:** 5 mg in 1-ml ampoule. **Tablet:** 2 mg; 5 mg.
Complementary List **[c]**	
chlorpromazine	***Injection:*** *25 mg (hydrochloride)/ml in 2-ml ampoule.* ***Oral liquid:*** *25 mg (hydrochloride)/5 ml.* ***Tablet:*** *10 mg; 25 mg; 50 mg; 100 mg (hydrochloride).*
haloperidol	***Injection:*** *5 mg in 1-ml ampoule.* ***Oral liquid:*** *2 mg/ml.* ***Solid oral dosage form:*** *0.5 mg; 2 mg; 5 mg.*

24.2 Medicines used in mood disorders

24.2.1 *Medicines used in depressive disorders*

□ amitriptyline	**Tablet:** 25 mg (hydrochloride).
fluoxetine	**Solid oral dosage form:** 20 mg (as hydrochloride).
Complementary List **[c]**	
fluoxetine [a]	***Solid oral dosage form:*** *20 mg (as hydrochloride).* [a] >8 years.

24.2.2 *Medicines used in bipolar disorders*

carbamazepine	**Tablet (scored):** 100 mg; 200 mg.
lithium carbonate	**Solid oral dosage form:** 300 mg.
valproic acid (sodium valproate)	**Tablet (enteric-coated):** 200 mg; 500 mg (sodium valproate).

24.3 Medicines for anxiety disorders

□ diazepam	**Tablet (scored):** 2 mg; 5 mg.

24. MEDICINES FOR MENTAL AND BEHAVIOURAL DISORDERS *(continued)*

24.4 Medicines used for obsessive compulsive disorders

clomipramine	**Capsule:** 10 mg; 25 mg (hydrochloride).

24.5 Medicines for disorders due to psychoactive substance use

nicotine replacement therapy (NRT)	**Chewing gum:** 2 mg; 4 mg (as polacrilex). **Transdermal patch:** 5 mg to 30 mg/16 hrs; 7 mg to 21 mg/24 hrs.
Complementary List	
□ *methadone**	***Concentrate for oral liquid:*** *5 mg/ml; 10 mg/ml (hydrochloride).* ***Oral liquid:*** *5 mg/5 ml; 10 mg/5 ml (hydrochloride).* * *The square box is added to include buprenorphine. The medicines should only be used within an established support programme.*

25. MEDICINES ACTING ON THE RESPIRATORY TRACT

25.1 Antiasthmatic and medicines for chronic obstructive pulmonary disease

□ beclometasone	**Inhalation (aerosol):** 50 micrograms (dipropionate) per dose; 100 micrograms (dipropionate) per dose (as CFC free forms).
□ budesonide [c]	**Inhalation (aerosol):** 100 micrograms per dose; 200 micrograms per dose.
epinephrine (adrenaline)	**Injection:** 1 mg (as hydrochloride **or** hydrogen tartrate) in 1-ml ampoule.
ipratropium bromide	**Inhalation (aerosol):** 20 micrograms/metered dose.
□ salbutamol	**Inhalation (aerosol):** 100 micrograms (as sulfate) per dose. **Injection:** 50 micrograms (as sulfate)/ml in 5-ml ampoule. **Metered dose inhaler (aerosol):** 100 micrograms (as sulfate) per dose. **Respirator solution for use in nebulizers:** 5 mg (as sulfate)/ml.

26. SOLUTIONS CORRECTING WATER, ELECTROLYTE AND ACID-BASE DISTURBANCES

26.1 Oral

oral rehydration salts	See section 17.5.1.

26. SOLUTIONS CORRECTING WATER, ELECTROLYTE AND ACID-BASE DISTURBANCES *(continued)*

potassium chloride	**Powder for solution.**

26.2 Parenteral

glucose	**Injectable solution:** 5% (isotonic); 10% (hypertonic); 50% (hypertonic).
glucose with sodium chloride	**Injectable solution:** 4% glucose, 0.18% sodium chloride (equivalent to Na+ 30 mmol/L, Cl- 30 mmol/L). **Injectable solution:** 5% glucose, 0.9% sodium chloride (equivalent to 150 mmol/L Na+ and 150 mmol/L Cl-); 5% glucose, 0.45% sodium chloride (equivalent to 75 mmol/L Na+ and 75 mmol/L Cl-) [c].
potassium chloride	**Solution:** 11.2% in 20-ml ampoule (equivalent to K+ 1.5 mmol/ml, Cl- 1.5 mmol/ml). **Solution for dilution:** 7.5% (equivalent to K 1 mmol/ml and Cl 1 mmol/ml) [c]; 15% (equivalent to K 2 mmol/ml and Cl 2 mmol/ml) [c].
sodium chloride	**Injectable solution:** 0.9% isotonic (equivalent to Na+ 154 mmol/L, Cl- 154 mmol/L).
sodium hydrogen carbonate	**Injectable solution:** 1.4% isotonic (equivalent to Na+ 167 mmol/L, HCO_3- 167 mmol/L). **Solution:** 8.4% in 10-ml ampoule (equivalent to Na+ 1000 mmol/L, HCO_3-1000 mmol/L).
□ sodium lactate, compound solution	**Injectable solution.**

26.3 Miscellaneous

water for injection	2-ml; 5-ml; 10-ml ampoules.

27. VITAMINS AND MINERALS

ascorbic acid	**Tablet:** 50 mg.
cholecalciferol* [c]	**Oral liquid:** 400 IU/ml. **Solid oral dosage form:** 400 IU; 1000 IU. * Ergocalciferol can be used as an alternative.
□ ergocalciferol	**Oral liquid:** 250 micrograms/ml (10 000 IU/ml). **Solid oral dosage form:** 1.25 mg (50 000 IU).

27. VITAMINS AND MINERALS *(continued)*	
iodine	**Capsule:** 200 mg. **Iodized oil:** 1 ml (480 mg iodine); 0.5 ml (240 mg iodine) in ampoule (oral **or** injectable); 0.57 ml (308 mg iodine) in dispenser bottle.
□ nicotinamide	**Tablet:** 50 mg.
pyridoxine	**Tablet:** 25 mg (hydrochloride).
retinol	**Capsule:** 50 000 IU; 100 000 IU; 200 000 IU (as palmitate). **Oral oily solution:** 100 000 IU (as palmitate)/ml in multidose dispenser. **Tablet (sugar-coated):** 10 000 IU (as palmitate). **Water-miscible injection:** 100 000 IU (as palmitate) in 2-ml ampoule.
riboflavin	**Tablet:** 5 mg.
sodium fluoride	In any appropriate topical formulation.
thiamine	**Tablet:** 50 mg (hydrochloride).
Complementary List	
calcium gluconate	***Injection:*** *100 mg/ml in 10-ml ampoule.*

28. EAR, NOSE AND THROAT CONDITIONS IN CHILDREN [c]	
acetic acid	**Topical:** 2%, in alcohol.
□ budesonide	**Nasal spray:** 100 micrograms per dose.
□ ciprofloxacin	**Topical:** 0.3% drops (as hydrochloride).
□ xylometazoline [a]	**Nasal spray:** 0.05%. [a] Not in children less than 3 months.

29. SPECIFIC MEDICINES FOR NEONATAL CARE [c]	
caffeine citrate	**Injection:** 20 mg/ml (equivalent to 10 mg caffeine base/ml). **Oral liquid:** 20 mg/ml (equivalent to 10 mg caffeine base/ml).
Complementary List	
□ *ibuprofen*	***Solution for injection:*** *5 mg/ml.*

29. SPECIFIC MEDICINES FOR NEONATAL CARE [c] *(continued)*	
□ *prostaglandin E*	***Solution for injection:*** ***Prostaglandin E1:*** *0.5 mg/ml in alcohol.* ***Prostaglandin E2:*** *1 mg/ml.*
surfactant	***Suspension for intratracheal instillation:*** *25 mg/ml* ***or*** *80 mg/ml.*

Table 1.1: Medicines with age or weight restrictions

atazanavir	>25 kg
atropine	>3 months
benzyl benzoate	>2 years
betamethasone topical preparations	Hydrocortisone preferred in neonates
cefazolin	>1 month
ceftriaxone	>41 weeks corrected gestational age
chlorphenamine	>1 year
diloxanide	>25 kg
doxycycline	>8 years (except for serious infections e.g. cholera)
efavirenz	>3 years or >10 kg
emtricitabine	>3 months
fluoxetine	>8 years
ibuprofen	>3 months (except IV form for patent *ductus arteriosus*)
mefloquine	>5 kg or >3 months
metoclopramide	Not in neonates
ondansetron	>1 month
saquinavir	>25 kg
silver sulfadiazine	>2 months
tetracaine	Not in preterm neonates
trimethoprim	>6 months
xylometazoline	>3 months

Table 1.2: Explanation of dosage forms

A. Principal dosage forms used in EML – Oral administration

Term	Definition
Solid oral dosage form	Refers to tablets or capsules or other solid dosage forms such as 'melts' that are immediate-release preparations. It implies that there is no difference in clinical efficacy or safety between the available dosage forms, and countries should therefore choose the form(s) to be listed depending on quality and availability. The term 'solid oral dosage form' is *never* intended to allow any type of modified-release tablet.
Tablets	Refers to: • uncoated or coated (film-coated or sugar-coated) tablets that are intended to be swallowed whole; • unscored and scored*; • tablets that are intended to be chewed before being swallowed; • tablets that are intended to be dispersed or dissolved in water or another suitable liquid before being swallowed; • tablets that are intended to be crushed before being swallowed. The term 'tablet' without qualification is *never* intended to allow any type of modified-release tablet.
Tablets (qualified)	Refers to a specific type of tablet: **chewable** – tablets that are intended to be chewed before being swallowed; **dispersible** – tablets that are intended to be dispersed in water or another suitable liquid before being swallowed; **soluble** – tablets that are intended to be dissolved in water or another suitable liquid before being swallowed; **crushable** – tablets that are intended to be crushed before being swallowed; **scored** – tablets bearing a break mark or marks where sub-division is intended in order to provide doses of less than one tablet; **sublingual** – tablets that are intended to be placed beneath the tongue.

continues

* Scored tablets may be divided for ease of swallowing, provided dose is a whole number of tablets.

continued

Term	Definition
	The term 'tablet' is *always* qualified with an additional term (in parentheses) in entries where one of the following types of tablet is intended: **gastro-resistant** (such tablets may sometimes be described as enteric-coated or as delayed-release), **prolonged-release** or another modified-release form.
Capsules	Refers to hard or soft capsules. The term 'capsule' without qualification is *never* intended to allow any type of modified-release capsule.
Capsules (qualified)	The term 'capsule' with qualification refers to **gastro-resistant** (such capsules may sometimes be described as enteric-coated or as delayed-release), **prolonged-release** or another modified-release form.
Granules	Preparations that are issued to patient as granules to be swallowed without further preparation, to be chewed, or to be taken in or with water or another suitable liquid. The term 'granules' without further qualification is *never* intended to allow any type of modified-release granules.
Oral powder	Preparations that are issued to patient as powder (usually as single-dose) to be taken in or with water or another suitable liquid.
Oral liquid	Liquid preparations intended to be *swallowed* i.e. oral solutions, suspensions, emulsions and oral drops, including those constituted from powders or granules, but *not* those preparations intended for *oromucosal* administration e.g. gargles and mouthwashes. Oral liquids presented as powders or granules may offer benefits in the form of better stability and lower transport costs. If more than one type of oral liquid is available on the same market (e.g. solution, suspension, granules for reconstitution), they may be interchanged and in such cases should be bioequivalent. It is preferable that oral liquids do not contain sugar and that solutions for children do not contain alcohol.

B. Principal dosage forms used in EMLc – Parenteral administration

Term	Definition
Injection	Refers to solutions, suspensions and emulsions including those constituted from powders or concentrated solutions.
Injection (qualified)	Route of administration is indicated in parentheses where relevant.
Injection (oily)	The term injection is qualified by (oily) in relevant entries.
Intravenous infusion	Refers to solutions and emulsions including those constituted from powders or concentrated solutions.

C. Other dosage forms

Mode of administration	Term to be used
To the eye	Eye drops, eye ointments.
Topical	For liquids: lotions, paints. For semi-solids: cream, ointment.
Rectal	Suppositories, gel or solution.
Vaginal	Pessaries or vaginal tablets.
Inhalation	Powder for inhalation, pressurized inhalation, nebulizer.

Annex 2

3rd WHO Model List of Essential Medicines for Children

Explanatory Notes

This Model List is intended for use for children up to 12 years of age.

The **Core List** presents a list of minimum medicine needs for a basic health-care system, listing the most efficacious, safe and cost-effective medicines for priority conditions. Priority conditions are selected on the basis of current and estimated future public health relevance, and potential for safe and cost-effective treatment.

The **Complementary List** presents essential medicines for priority diseases, for which specialized diagnostic or monitoring facilities, and/or specialist medical care, and/or specialist training are needed. In case of doubt medicines may also be listed as complementary on the basis of consistent higher costs or less attractive cost-effectiveness in a variety of settings.

The **square box symbol** (□) is primarily intended to indicate similar clinical performance within a pharmacological class. The listed medicine should be the example of the class for which there is the best evidence for effectiveness and safety. In some cases, this may be the first medicine that is licensed for marketing; in other instances, subsequently licensed compounds may be safer or more effective. Where there is no difference in terms of efficacy and safety data, the listed medicine should be the one that is generally available at the lowest price, based on international drug price information sources.

Therapeutic equivalence is only indicated on the basis of reviews of efficacy and safety and when consistent with WHO clinical guidelines. National lists should not use a similar symbol and should be specific in their final selection, which would depend on local availability and price.

The format and numbering of the 17th WHO Model List of Essential Medicines have been retained but, as indicated in the text, some sections have been deleted because they contain medicines that are not relevant for children.

[a] indicates that there is an age or weight restriction on use of the medicines; the details for each medicine are in Table 1.1, Annex 1.

In the List of Essential Medicines for Children, an additional symbol is used:

[R] indicates that the Committee has endorsed the medicine as essential but has requested a review of the efficacy and safety to confirm this decision, or to expand use to additional age groups.

The presence of an entry on the Essential Medicines List carries no assurance as to pharmaceutical quality. It is the responsibility of the relevant national or regional drug regulatory authority to ensure that each product is of appropriate pharmaceutical quality (including stability) and that when relevant, different products are interchangeable.

For recommendations and advice concerning all aspects of the quality assurance of medicines see the WHO Medicines web site http://www.who.int/medicines/areas/quality_assurance/en/index.html.

Medicines and dosage forms are listed in alphabetical order within each section and there is no implication of preference for one form over another. Standard treatment guidelines should be consulted for information on appropriate dosage forms.

The main terms used for dosage forms in the Essential Medicines List can be found in Table 1.2, Annex 1.

Definitions of many of these terms and pharmaceutical quality requirements applicable to the different categories are published in the current edition of *The International Pharmacopoeia* http://www.who.int/medicines/publications/pharmacopoeia/en/index.html.

1. ANAESTHETICS

1.1 General anaesthetics and oxygen

1.1.1 *Inhalational medicines*

halothane	**Inhalation.**
isoflurane	**Inhalation.**
nitrous oxide	**Inhalation.**
oxygen	**Inhalation** (medicinal gas).

1.1.2 *Injectable medicines*

ketamine	**Injection:** 50 mg (as hydrochloride)/ml in 10-ml vial.
propofol*	**Injection:** 10 mg/ml; 20 mg/ml. * Thiopental may be used as an alternative depending on local availability and cost.

1.2 Local anaesthetics

☐ bupivacaine	**Injection:** 0.25%; 0.5% (hydrochloride) in vial. **Injection for spinal anaesthesia:** 0.5% (hydrochloride) in 4-ml ampoule to be mixed with 7.5% glucose solution.
☐ lidocaine	**Injection:** 1%; 2% (hydrochloride) in vial. **Injection for spinal anaesthesia:** 5% (hydrochloride) in 2-ml ampoule to be mixed with 7.5% glucose solution. **Topical forms:** 2% to 4% (hydrochloride).
lidocaine + epinephrine (adrenaline)	**Dental cartridge:** 2% (hydrochloride) + epinephrine 1:80 000. **Injection:** 1%; 2% (hydrochloride **or** sulfate) + epinephrine 1:200 000 in vial.

1.3 Preoperative medication and sedation for short-term procedures

atropine	**Injection:** 1 mg (sulfate) in 1-ml ampoule.
☐ midazolam	**Injection:** 1 mg/ml. **Oral liquid:** 2 mg/ml. **Tablet:** 7.5 mg; 15 mg.
morphine	**Injection:** 10 mg (sulfate **or** hydrochloride) in 1-ml ampoule.

2. ANALGESICS, ANTIPYRETICS, NON-STEROIDAL ANTI-INFLAMMATORY MEDICINES (NSAIMs), MEDICINES USED TO TREAT GOUT AND DISEASE-MODIFYING AGENTS IN RHEUMATOID DISORDERS (DMARDs)

2.1 Non-opioids and non-steroidal anti-inflammatory medicines (NSAIMs)

ibuprofen [a]	**Oral liquid:** 200 mg/5 ml. **Tablet:** 200 mg; 400 mg. [a] >3 months.
paracetamol*	**Oral liquid:** 125 mg/5 ml. **Suppository:** 100 mg. **Tablet:** 100 mg to 500 mg. * Not recommended for anti-inflammatory use due to lack of proven benefit to that effect.
Complementary List	
*acetylsalicylic acid**	***Suppository:*** *50 mg to 150 mg.* ***Tablet:*** *100 mg to 500 mg.* * *For use for rheumatic fever, juvenile arthritis, Kawasaki disease.*

2.2 Opioid analgesics

morphine	**Injection:** 10 mg (morphine hydrochloride **or** morphine sulfate) in 1-ml ampoule. **Oral liquid:** 10 mg (morphine hydrochloride **or** morphine sulfate)/5 ml. **Tablet:** 10 mg (morphine sulfate). **Tablet (prolonged release):** 10 mg; 30 mg; 60 mg (morphine sulfate).

~~2.3 Medicines used to treat gout~~

2.4 Disease-modifying agents used in rheumatoid disorders (DMARDs)

Complementary List	
hydroxychloroquine	***Solid oral dosage form:*** *200 mg (as sulfate).*
methotrexate	***Tablet:*** *2.5 mg (as sodium salt).*

3. ANTIALLERGICS AND MEDICINES USED IN ANAPHYLAXIS

□ chlorphenamine [a] [R]	**Injection:** 10 mg (hydrogen maleate) in 1-ml ampoule. **Oral liquid:** 2 mg/5 ml (hydrogen maleate). **Tablet:** 4 mg (hydrogen maleate). [a] >1 year. [R] Review of diphenhydramine to assess comparative efficacy and safety with chlorphenamine as a possible preferable alternative.
dexamethasone	**Injection:** 4 mg/ml in 1-ml ampoule (as disodium phosphate salt).
epinephrine (adrenaline)	**Injection:** 1 mg (as hydrochloride **or** hydrogen tartrate) in 1-ml ampoule.
hydrocortisone	**Powder for injection:** 100 mg (as sodium succinate) in vial.
□ prednisolone	**Oral liquid:** 5 mg/ml. **Tablet:** 5 mg; 25 mg.

4. ANTIDOTES AND OTHER SUBSTANCES USED IN POISONINGS

4.1 Non-specific

charcoal, activated	**Powder.**

4.2 Specific

acetylcysteine	**Injection:** 200 mg/ml in 10-ml ampoule. **Oral liquid:** 10%; 20%.
atropine	**Injection:** 1 mg (sulfate) in 1-ml ampoule.
calcium gluconate	**Injection:** 100 mg/ml in 10-ml ampoule.
naloxone	**Injection:** 400 micrograms (hydrochloride) in 1-ml ampoule.
Complementary List	
deferoxamine	***Powder for injection:*** *500 mg (mesilate) in vial.*
dimercaprol	***Injection in oil:*** *50 mg/ml in 2-ml ampoule.*
sodium calcium edetate	***Injection:*** *200 mg/ml in 5-ml ampoule.*
succimer	***Solid oral dosage form:*** *100 mg.*

5. ANTICONVULSANTS/ANTIEPILEPTICS

carbamazepine	**Oral liquid:** 100 mg/5 ml. **Tablet (chewable):** 100 mg; 200 mg. **Tablet (scored):** 100 mg; 200 mg.
diazepam	**Gel or rectal solution:** 5 mg/ml in 0.5-ml; 2-ml; 4-ml tubes.
□ lorazepam	**Parenteral formulation:** 2 mg/ml in 1-ml ampoule; 4 mg/ml in 1-ml ampoule.
phenobarbital	**Injection:** 200 mg/ml (sodium). **Oral liquid:** 15 mg/5 ml. **Tablet:** 15 mg to 100 mg.
phenytoin	**Injection:** 50 mg/ml in 5-ml vial (sodium salt). **Oral liquid:** 25 mg to 30 mg/5 ml.* **Solid oral dosage form:** 25 mg; 50 mg; 100 mg (sodium salt). **Tablet (chewable):** 50 mg. * The presence of both 25 mg/5 ml and 30 mg/5 ml strengths on the same market would cause confusion in prescribing and dispensing and should be avoided.
valproic acid (sodium valproate)	**Oral liquid:** 200 mg/5 ml. **Tablet (crushable):** 100 mg. **Tablet (enteric-coated):** 200 mg; 500 mg (sodium valproate).
Complementary List	
ethosuximide	***Capsule:*** *250 mg.* ***Oral liquid:*** *250 mg/5 ml.*

6. ANTI-INFECTIVE MEDICINES

6.1 Anthelminthics

6.1.1 *Intestinal anthelminthics*

albendazole	**Tablet (chewable):** 400 mg.
levamisole*	**Tablet:** 50 mg; 150 mg (as hydrochloride). * The Expert Committee recommended that this medicine be reviewed for deletion at its next meeting. Should only be used in combination with other anthelminthics.
mebendazole	**Tablet (chewable):** 100 mg; 500 mg.

6. ANTI-INFECTIVE MEDICINES *(continued)*

niclosamide*	**Tablet (chewable):** 500 mg. * Niclosamide is listed for use when praziquantel treatment fails. The Expert Committee recommended that this medicine be reviewed for deletion at its next meeting.
praziquantel	**Tablet:** 150 mg; 600 mg.
pyrantel	**Oral liquid:** 50 mg (as embonate **or** pamoate)/ml. **Tablet (chewable):** 250 mg (as embonate **or** pamoate).

6.1.2 *Antifilarials*

albendazole	**Tablet (chewable):** 400 mg.
diethylcarbamazine	**Tablet:** 50 mg; 100 mg (dihydrogen citrate).
ivermectin	**Tablet (scored):** 3 mg; 6 mg.

6.1.3 *Antischistosomals and other antitrematode medicines*

praziquantel	**Tablet:** 600 mg.
triclabendazole	**Tablet:** 250 mg.
Complementary List	
*oxamniquine**	***Capsule:** 250 mg.* ***Oral liquid:** 250 mg/5 ml.* * *Oxamniquine is listed for use when praziquantel treatment fails.*

6.2 Antibacterials

6.2.1 *Beta Lactam medicines*

amoxicillin	**Powder for oral liquid:** 125 mg (as trihydrate)/5 ml; 250 mg (as trihydrate)/5 ml. **Solid oral dosage form:** 250 mg; 500 mg (as trihydrate).
amoxicillin + clavulanic acid	**Oral liquid:** 125 mg amoxicillin + 31.25 mg clavulanic acid/5 ml AND 250 mg amoxicillin + 62.5 mg clavulanic acid/5 ml. **Tablet:** 500 mg (as trihydrate) + 125 mg (as potassium salt).
ampicillin	**Powder for injection:** 500 mg; 1 g (as sodium salt) in vial.
benzathine benzylpenicillin	**Powder for injection:** 900 mg benzylpenicillin (= 1.2 million IU) in 5-ml vial; 1.44 g benzylpenicillin (= 2.4 million IU) in 5-ml vial.

6. ANTI-INFECTIVE MEDICINES *(continued)*

benzylpenicillin	**Powder for injection:** 600 mg (= 1 million IU); 3 g (= 5 million IU) (sodium **or** potassium salt) in vial.
cefalexin	**Powder for reconstitution with water:** 125 mg/5 ml; 250 mg/5 ml (anhydrous). **Solid oral dosage form:** 250 mg (as monohydrate).
□ cefazolin* [a]	**Powder for injection:** 1 g (as sodium salt) in vial. * For surgical prophylaxis. [a] >1 month.
ceftriaxone* [a]	**Powder for injection:** 250 mg; 1 g (as sodium salt) in vial. * Do not administer with calcium and avoid in infants with hyperbilirubinemia. [a] >41 weeks corrected gestational age.
□ cloxacillin	**Capsule:** 500 mg; 1 g (as sodium salt). **Powder for injection:** 500 mg (as sodium salt) in vial. **Powder for oral liquid:** 125 mg (as sodium salt)/5 ml.
phenoxymethylpenicillin	**Powder for oral liquid:** 250 mg (as potassium salt)/5 ml. **Tablet:** 250 mg (as potassium salt).
procaine benzylpenicillin*	**Powder for injection:** 1 g (=1 million IU); 3 g (=3 million IU) in vial. * Procaine benzylpenicillin is not recommended as first-line treatment for neonatal sepsis except in settings with high neonatal mortality, when given by trained health workers in cases where hospital care is not achievable.
Complementary List	
*cefotaxime**	***Powder for injection:** 250 mg per vial (as sodium salt).* * *3rd generation cephalosporin of choice for use in hospitalized neonates.*
ceftazidime	***Powder for injection:** 250 mg **or** 1 g (as pentahydrate) in vial.*
imipenem + cilastatin**	***Powder for injection:** 250 mg (as monohydrate) + 250 mg (as sodium salt); 500 mg (as monohydrate) + 500 mg (as sodium salt) in vial.* * *Only listed for the treatment of life-threatening hospital-based infection due to suspected or proven multidrug-resistant infection. Meropenem is indicated for the treatment of meningitis and is licensed for use in children over the age of 3 months.*

6. ANTI-INFECTIVE MEDICINES *(continued)*

6.2.2 *Other antibacterials*

azithromycin*	**Capsule:** 250 mg; 500 mg (anhydrous). **Oral liquid:** 200 mg/5 ml. * Only listed for trachoma.
chloramphenicol	**Capsule:** 250 mg. **Oily suspension for injection*:** 0.5 g (as sodium succinate)/ml in 2-ml ampoule. * Only for the presumptive treatment of epidemic meningitis in children older than 2 years. **Oral liquid:** 150 mg (as palmitate)/5 ml. **Powder for injection:** 1 g (sodium succinate) in vial.
ciprofloxacin	**Oral liquid:** 250 mg/5 ml (anhydrous). **Solution for IV infusion:** 2 mg/ml (as hyclate). **Tablet:** 250 mg (as hydrochloride).
doxycycline [a]	**Oral liquid:** 25 mg/5 ml; 50 mg/5 ml (anhydrous). **Solid oral dosage form:** 50 mg; 100 mg (as hyclate). [a] Use in children <8 years only for life-threatening infections when no alternative exists.
erythromycin	**Powder for oral liquid:** 125 mg/5 ml (as stearate **or** estolate **or** ethyl succinate). **Solid oral dosage form:** 250 mg (as stearate **or** estolate **or** ethyl succinate).
□ gentamicin	**Injection:** 10 mg; 40 mg (as sulfate)/ml in 2-ml vial.
metronidazole	**Injection:** 500 mg in 100-ml vial. **Oral liquid:** 200 mg (as benzoate)/5 ml. **Tablet:** 200 mg to 500 mg.
nitrofurantoin	**Oral liquid:** 25 mg/5 ml. **Tablet:** 100 mg.
sulfamethoxazole + trimethoprim	**Injection:** 80 mg + 16 mg/ml in 5-ml ampoule; 80 mg + 16 mg/ml in 10-ml ampoule. **Oral liquid:** 200 mg + 40 mg/5 ml. **Tablet:** 100 mg + 20 mg; 400 mg + 80 mg.
trimethoprim [a]	**Oral liquid:** 50 mg/5 ml. **Tablet:** 100 mg; 200 mg. [a] >6 months.

6. ANTI-INFECTIVE MEDICINES *(continued)*

Complementary List

clindamycin	***Capsule:*** *150 mg (as hydrochloride).* ***Injection:*** *150 mg (as phosphate)/ml.* ***Oral liquid:*** *75 mg/5 ml (as palmitate).*
vancomycin	***Powder for injection:*** *250 mg (as hydrochloride) in vial.*

6.2.3 *Antileprosy medicines*

Medicines used in the treatment of leprosy should never be used except in combination. Combination therapy is essential to prevent the emergence of drug resistance. Colour coded blister packs (MDT blister packs) containing standard two-medicine (paucibacillary leprosy) or three-medicine (multibacillary leprosy) combinations for adult and childhood leprosy should be used. MDT blister packs can be supplied free of charge through WHO.

clofazimine	**Capsule:** 50 mg; 100 mg.
dapsone	**Tablet:** 25 mg; 50 mg; 100 mg.
rifampicin	**Solid oral dosage form:** 150 mg; 300 mg.

6.2.4 *Antituberculosis medicines*

The Committee recommends and endorses the use of fixed-dose combinations and the development of appropriate new fixed-dose combinations, including modified dosage forms, non-refrigerated products and paediatric dosage forms of assured pharmaceutical quality.

ethambutol	**Oral liquid:** 25 mg/ml. **Tablet:** 100 mg; 400 mg (hydrochloride).
isoniazid	**Oral liquid:** 50 mg/5 ml. **Tablet:** 100 mg to 300 mg. **Tablet (scored):** 50 mg.
pyrazinamide	**Oral liquid:** 30 mg/ml. **Tablet:** 400 mg. **Tablet (dispersible):** 150 mg. **Tablet (scored):** 150 mg.
rifampicin	**Oral liquid:** 20 mg/ml. **Solid oral dosage form:** 150 mg; 300 mg.
streptomycin R	**Powder for injection:** 1 g (as sulfate) in vial. R Review of safety and efficacy of streptomycin in childhood TB.

6. ANTI-INFECTIVE MEDICINES *(continued)*

Complementary List

Reserve second-line drugs for the treatment of multidrug-resistant tuberculosis (MDR-TB) should be used in specialized centres adhering to WHO standards for TB control. R

R The Committee requests a review of the medicines for MDR-TB in children.

amikacin	***Powder for injection:*** *100 mg; 500 mg; 1 g (as sulfate) in vial.*
capreomycin	***Powder for injection:*** *1 g (as sulfate) in vial.*
cycloserine	***Solid oral dosage form:*** *250 mg.*
ethionamide	***Tablet:*** *125 mg; 250 mg.*
kanamycin	***Powder for injection:*** *1 g (as sulfate) in vial.*
*ofloxacin**	***Tablet:*** *200 mg; 400 mg.* * *Levofloxacin may be an alternative based on availability and programme considerations.*
p-aminosalicylic acid	***Granules:*** *4 g in sachet.* ***Tablet:*** *500 mg.*

6.3 Antifungal medicines

fluconazole	**Capsule:** 50 mg. **Injection:** 2 mg/ml in vial. **Oral liquid:** 50 mg/5 ml.
griseofulvin	**Oral liquid:** 125 mg/5 ml. **Solid oral dosage form:** 125 mg; 250 mg.
nystatin	**Lozenge:** 100 000 IU. **Oral liquid:** 50 mg/5 ml; 100 000 IU/ml. **Tablet:** 100 000 IU; 500 000 IU.

Complementary List

amphotericin B	***Powder for injection:*** *50 mg in vial.* *As sodium deoxycholate **or** liposomal complex.*
flucytosine	***Capsule:*** *250 mg.* ***Infusion:*** *2.5 g in 250 ml.*
potassium iodide	***Saturated solution.***

6. ANTI-INFECTIVE MEDICINES *(continued)*

6.4 Antiviral medicines

6.4.1 *Antiherpes medicines*

aciclovir	**Oral liquid:** 200 mg/5 ml. **Powder for injection:** 250 mg (as sodium salt) in vial. **Tablet:** 200 mg.

6.4.2 *Antiretrovirals*

Based on current evidence and experience of use, medicines in the following three classes of antiretrovirals are included as essential medicines for treatment and prevention of HIV (prevention of mother-to-child transmission and post-exposure prophylaxis). The Committee emphasizes the importance of using these products in accordance with global and national guidelines. The Committee recommends and endorses the use of fixed-dose combinations and the development of appropriate new fixed-dose combinations, including modified dosage forms, non-refrigerated products and paediatric dosage forms of assured pharmaceutical quality.

Scored tablets can be used in children and therefore can be considered for inclusion in the listing of tablets, provided adequate quality products are available.

6.4.2.1 *Nucleoside/Nucleotide reverse transcriptase inhibitors*

abacavir (ABC)	**Oral liquid:** 100 mg (as sulfate)/5 ml. **Tablet:** 300 mg (as sulfate).
didanosine (ddI)	**Buffered powder for oral liquid:** 100-mg; 167-mg; 250-mg packets. **Capsule (unbuffered enteric-coated):** 125 mg; 200 mg; 250 mg; 400 mg. **Tablet (buffered chewable, dispersible):** 25 mg; 50 mg; 100 mg; 150 mg; 200 mg.
emtricitabine (FTC)* [a]	**Capsule:** 200 mg. **Oral liquid:** 10 mg/ml. * FTC is an acceptable alternative to 3TC, based on knowledge of the pharmacology, the resistance patterns and clinical trials of antiretrovirals. [a] >3 months.
lamivudine (3TC)	**Oral liquid:** 50 mg/5 ml. **Tablet:** 150 mg.
stavudine (d4T)	**Capsule:** 15 mg; 20 mg; 30 mg. **Powder for oral liquid:** 5 mg/5 ml.

6. ANTI-INFECTIVE MEDICINES *(continued)*

zidovudine (ZDV **or** AZT)	**Capsule:** 100 mg; 250 mg. **Oral liquid:** 50 mg/5 ml. **Solution for IV infusion injection:** 10 mg/ml in 20-ml vial. **Tablet:** 300 mg.

6.4.2.2 *Non-nucleoside reverse transcriptase inhibitors*

efavirenz (EFV **or** EFZ) [a]	**Capsule:** 50 mg; 100 mg; 200 mg. **Oral liquid:** 150 mg/5 ml. **Tablet:** 600 mg. [a] >3 years **or** >10 kg.
nevirapine (NVP)	**Oral liquid:** 50 mg/5 ml. **Tablet:** 200 mg.

6.4.2.3 *Protease inhibitors*

Selection of protease inhibitor(s) from the Model List will need to be determined by each country after consideration of international and national treatment guidelines and experience. Ritonavir is recommended for use in combination as a pharmacological booster, and not as an antiretroviral in its own right. All other protease inhibitors should be used in boosted forms (e.g. with ritonavir).

atazanavir [a]	**Solid oral dosage form:** 100 mg; 150 mg; 300 mg (as sulfate). [a] >25 kg.
lopinavir + ritonavir (LPV/r)	**Capsule:** 133.3 mg + 33.3 mg. **Oral liquid:** 400 mg + 100 mg/5 ml. **Tablet (heat stable):** 100 mg + 25 mg; 200 mg + 50 mg.
ritonavir	**Oral liquid:** 400 mg/5 ml. **Solid oral dosage form:** 100 mg. **Tablet (heat stable):** 25 mg; 100 mg.
saquinavir (SQV) [a]	**Solid oral dosage form:** 200 mg (as mesilate). [a] >25 kg.

FIXED-DOSE COMBINATIONS

lamivudine + nevirapine + stavudine	**Tablet:** 150 mg + 200 mg + 30 mg. **Tablet (dispersible):** 30 mg + 50 mg + 6 mg; 60 mg + 100 mg + 12 mg.

6. ANTI-INFECTIVE MEDICINES *(continued)*

lamivudine + nevirapine + zidovudine	**Tablet:** 30 mg + 50 mg + 60 mg; 150 mg + 200 mg + 300 mg.
lamivudine + zidovudine	**Tablet:** 30 mg + 60 mg; 150 mg + 300 mg.

6.4.3 *Other antivirals*

oseltamivir*	**Capsule:** 30 mg; 45 mg; 75 mg (as phosphate). **Oral powder:** 12 mg/ml. * Oseltamivir should be used only in compliance with the WHO treatment guidelines, i.e. (1) for treatment of patients with severe or progressive clinical illness with confirmed or suspected influenza pandemic (H1N1) 2009, (2) for the treatment of patients with confirmed or suspected but uncomplicated illness due to pandemic influenza virus infection who were in higher risk groups, most notably for pregnant women and children under 2 years of age.
ribavirin*	**Injection for intravenous administration:** 800 mg and 1 g in 10-ml phosphate buffer solution. **Solid oral dosage form:** 200 mg; 400 mg; 600 mg. * For the treatment of viral haemorrhagic fevers only.

6.5 Antiprotozoal medicines

6.5.1 *Antiamoebic and antigiardiasis medicines*

diloxanide [a]	**Tablet:** 500 mg (furoate). [a] >25 kg.
□ metronidazole	**Injection:** 500 mg in 100-ml vial. **Oral liquid:** 200 mg (as benzoate)/5 ml. **Tablet:** 200 mg to 500 mg.

6.5.2 *Antileishmaniasis medicines*

amphotericin B	**Powder for injection:** 50 mg in vial. As sodium deoxycholate **or** liposomal complex.
miltefosine	**Solid oral dosage form:** 10 mg; 50 mg.
paromomycin	**Solution for intramuscular injection:** 750 mg of paromomycin base (as the sulfate).
sodium stibogluconate **or** meglumine antimoniate [R]	**Injection:** 100 mg/ml, 1 vial = 30 ml **or** 30%, equivalent to approximately 8.1% antimony (pentavalent) in 5-ml ampoule. [R] Review of comparative effectiveness and safety of antimonials for leishmaniasis, and whether they should be kept on the Core List or moved to the Complementary List.

6. ANTI-INFECTIVE MEDICINES *(continued)*

6.5.3 *Antimalarial medicines*

6.5.3.1 *For curative treatment*

Medicines for the treatment of *P. falciparum* malaria cases should be used in combination. The list currently recommends combinations according to treatment guidelines. The Committee recognizes that not all of these FDCs exist and encourages their development and rigorous testing. The Committee also encourages development and testing of rectal dosage formulations.

amodiaquine*	**Tablet:** 153 mg **or** 200 mg (as hydrochloride). * To be used in combination with artesunate 50 mg.
artemether*	**Oily injection:** 80 mg/ml in 1-ml ampoule. * For use in the management of severe malaria.
artemether + lumefantrine*	**Tablet:** 20 mg + 120 mg. **Tablet (dispersible):** 20 mg + 120 mg. * Not recommended in the first trimester of pregnancy or in children below 5 kg.
artesunate*	**Injection:** ampoules, containing 60 mg anhydrous artesunic acid with a separate ampoule of 5% sodium bicarbonate solution. For use in the management of severe malaria. **Rectal dosage form:** 50 mg; 200 mg capsules (for pre-referral treatment of severe malaria only; patients should be taken to an appropriate health facility for follow-up care). **Tablet:** 50 mg. * To be used in combination with either amodiaquine, mefloquine **or** sulfadoxine + pyrimethamine.
artesunate + amodiaquine*	**Tablet:** 25 mg + 67.5 mg; 50 mg + 135 mg; 100 mg + 270 mg. * Other combinations that deliver the target doses required such as 153 mg **or** 200 mg (as hydrochloride) with 50 mg artesunate can be alternatives.
chloroquine*	**Oral liquid:** 50 mg (as phosphate **or** sulfate)/5 ml. **Tablet:** 100 mg; 150 mg (as phosphate **or** sulfate). * For use only for the treatment of *P. vivax* infection.
doxycycline*	**Capsule:** 100 mg (as hydrochloride **or** hyclate). **Tablet (dispersible):** 100 mg (as monohydrate). * For use only in combination with quinine.

6. ANTI-INFECTIVE MEDICINES *(continued)*	
mefloquine*	**Tablet:** 250 mg (as hydrochloride). * To be used in combination with artesunate 50 mg.
primaquine*	**Tablet:** 7.5 mg; 15 mg (as diphosphate). * Only for use to achieve radical cure of *P. vivax* and *P. ovale* infections, given for 14 days.
quinine*	**Injection:** 300 mg quinine hydrochloride/ml in 2-ml ampoule. **Tablet:** 300 mg (quinine sulfate) **or** 300 mg (quinine bisulfate). * For use only in the management of severe malaria, and should be used in combination with doxycycline.
sulfadoxine + pyrimethamine*	**Tablet:** 500 mg + 25 mg. * Only in combination with artesunate 50 mg.
6.5.3.2 *For prophylaxis*	
chloroquine*	**Oral liquid:** 50 mg (as phosphate **or** sulfate)/5 ml. **Tablet:** 150 mg (as phosphate **or** sulfate). * For use only for the treatment of *P. vivax* infection.
doxycycline [a]	**Solid oral dosage form:** 100 mg (as hydrochloride **or** hyclate). [a] >8 years.
mefloquine [a]	**Tablet:** 250 mg (as hydrochloride). [a] >5 kg **or** >3 months.
proguanil*	**Tablet:** 100 mg (as hydrochloride). * For use only in combination with chloroquine.
6.5.4 *Antipneumocystosis and antitoxoplasmosis medicines*	
pyrimethamine	**Tablet:** 25 mg.
sulfadiazine	**Tablet:** 500 mg.
sulfamethoxazole + trimethoprim	**Injection:** 80 mg + 16 mg/ml in 5-ml ampoule; 80 mg + 16 mg/ml in 10-ml ampoule. **Oral liquid:** 200 mg + 40 mg/5 ml. **Tablet:** 100 mg + 20 mg; 400 mg + 80 mg.

6. ANTI-INFECTIVE MEDICINES *(continued)*

6.5.5 *Antitrypanosomal medicines*

6.5.5.1 *African trypanosomiasis*

Medicines for the treatment of 1st stage African trypanosomiasis.

pentamidine*	**Powder for injection:** 200 mg (as isetionate) in vial. * To be used for the treatment of *Trypanosoma brucei gambiense* infection.
suramin sodium*	**Powder for injection:** 1 g in vial. * To be used for the treatment of the initial phase of *Trypanosoma brucei rhodesiense* infection.

Medicines for the treatment of 2nd stage African trypanosomiasis

eflornithine*	**Injection:** 200 mg (hydrochloride)/ml in 100-ml bottle. * To be used for the treatment of *Trypanosoma brucei gambiense* infection.
Complementary List	
melarsoprol	***Injection:** 3.6% solution in 5-ml ampoule (180 mg of active compound).*

6.5.5.2 *American trypanosomiasis* R

benznidazole	**Tablet:** 100 mg.
nifurtimox	**Tablet:** 30 mg; 120 mg; 250 mg.

7. ANTIMIGRAINE MEDICINES

7.1 For treatment of acute attack

ibuprofen	**Tablet:** 200 mg; 400 mg.
paracetamol	**Oral liquid:** 125 mg/5 ml. **Tablet:** 300 mg to 500 mg.

7.2 For prophylaxis

propranolol	**Tablet:** 20 mg; 40 mg (hydrochloride).

8. ANTINEOPLASTIC, IMMUNOSUPPRESSIVES AND MEDICINES USED IN PALLIATIVE CARE

8.1 Immunosuppressive medicines

Complementary List

azathioprine	***Powder for injection:*** *100 mg (as sodium salt) in vial.* ***Tablet (scored):*** *50 mg.*
ciclosporin	***Capsule:*** *25 mg.* ***Concentrate for injection:*** *50 mg/ml in 1-ml ampoule for organ transplantation.*

8.2 Cytotoxic and adjuvant medicines

Medicines listed below should be used according to protocols for treatment of the diseases.

Complementary List

ACUTE LYMPHOBLASTIC LEUKAEMIA

STEP 1

asparaginase	***Powder for injection:*** *10 000 IU in vial.*
dexamethasone	***Oral liquid:*** *2 mg/5 ml.*
mercaptopurine	***Tablet:*** *50 mg.*
methotrexate	***Powder for injection:*** *50 mg (as sodium salt) in vial.* ***Tablet:*** *2.5 mg (as sodium salt).*
methylprednisolone	***Injection:*** *40 mg/ml (as sodium succinate) in 1-ml single dose vial and 5-ml multidose vials; 80 mg/ml (as sodium succinate) in 1-ml single dose vial.*
prednisolone	***Oral liquid:*** *5 mg/ml.*
vincristine	***Powder for injection:*** *1 mg; 5 mg (sulfate) in vial.*

STEP 2

cyclophosphamide	***Powder for injection:*** *500 mg in vial.*
cytarabine	***Powder for injection:*** *100 mg in vial.*
daunorubicin	***Powder for injection:*** *50 mg (hydrochloride) in vial.*
doxorubicin	***Powder for injection:*** *10 mg; 50 mg (hydrochloride) in vial.*
hydrocortisone	***Powder for injection:*** *100 mg (as sodium succinate) in vial.*

8. ANTINEOPLASTIC, IMMUNOSUPPRESSIVES AND MEDICINES USED IN PALLIATIVE CARE *(continued)*

methotrexate	***Powder for injection:*** *50 mg (as sodium salt) in vial.*
thioguanine	***Solid oral dosage form:*** *40 mg.*
WILMS' TUMOUR (NEPHROBLASTOMA)	
STEP 1 & STEP 2	
dactinomycin	***Powder for injection:*** *500 micrograms in vial.*
daunorubicin	***Powder for injection:*** *50 mg (hydrochloride) in vial.*
vincristine	***Powder for injection:*** *1 mg; 5 mg (sulfate) in vial.*
BURKITT'S LYMPHOMA	
STEP 1 & STEP 2	
cyclophosphamide	***Powder for injection:*** *500 mg in vial.*
cytarabine	***Powder for injection:*** *100 mg in vial.*
doxorubicin	***Powder for injection:*** *10 mg; 50 mg (hydrochloride) in vial.*
prednisolone	***Oral liquid:*** *5 mg/ml.*
vincristine	***Powder for injection:*** *1 mg; 5 mg (sulfate) in vial.*
ADJUVANT MEDICINES	
allopurinol	***Tablet:*** *100 mg; 300 mg.*
mesna	***Injection:*** *100 mg/ml in 4-ml and 10-ml ampoules.* ***Tablet:*** *400 mg; 600 mg.*

~~8.3 Hormones and antihormones~~

8.4 Medicines used in palliative care

amitriptyline	**Tablet:** 10 mg; 25 mg.
cyclizine	**Injection:** 50 mg/ml. **Tablet:** 50 mg.
dexamethasone	**Injection:** 4 mg/ml in 1-ml ampoule (as disodium phosphate salt). **Tablet:** 2 mg.

8. ANTINEOPLASTIC, IMMUNOSUPPRESSIVES AND MEDICINES USED IN PALLIATIVE CARE *(continued)*

diazepam	**Injection:** 5 mg/ml. **Oral liquid:** 2 mg/5 ml. **Rectal solution:** 2.5 mg; 5 mg; 10 mg. **Tablet:** 5 mg; 10 mg.
docusate sodium	**Capsule:** 100 mg. **Oral liquid:** 50 mg/5 ml.
fluoxetine [a]	**Solid oral dosage form:** 20 mg (as hydrochloride). [a] >8 years.
hyoscine hydrobromide	**Injection:** 400 micrograms/ml; 600 micrograms/ml. **Transdermal patches:** 1 mg/72 hours.
ibuprofen [a]	**Oral liquid:** 200 mg/5 ml. **Tablet:** 200 mg; 400 mg; 600 mg. [a] Not in children less than 3 months.
lactulose	**Oral liquid:** 3.1–3.7 g/5 ml.
midazolam	**Injection:** 1 mg/ml; 5 mg/ml.
morphine	**Granules (modified release) (to mix with water):** 20 mg; 30 mg; 60 mg; 100 mg; 200 mg. **Injection:** 10 mg/ml. **Oral liquid:** 10 mg/5 ml. **Tablet (controlled release):** 10 mg; 30 mg; 60 mg. **Tablet (immediate release):** 10 mg.
ondansetron [a]	**Injection:** 2 mg base/ml in 2-ml ampoule (as hydrochloride). **Oral liquid:** 4 mg base/ 5 ml. **Solid oral dosage form:** Eq 4 mg base; Eq 8 mg base. [a] >1 month.
senna	**Oral liquid:** 7.5 mg/5 ml.

~~9. ANTIPARKINSONISM MEDICINES~~

10. MEDICINES AFFECTING THE BLOOD

10.1 Antianaemia medicines R

R The Committee proposed a review of the evidence for appropriate dose combinations of iron and folic acid for children.

ferrous salt	**Oral liquid:** equivalent to 25 mg iron (as sulfate)/ml. **Tablet:** equivalent to 60 mg iron.
folic acid	**Tablet:** 1 mg; 5 mg.
hydroxocobalamin	**Injection:** 1 mg (as acetate, hydrochloride **or** as sulfate) in 1-ml ampoule.

10.2 Medicines affecting coagulation

phytomenadione	**Injection:** 1 mg/ml; 10 mg/ml in 5-ml ampoule. **Tablet:** 10 mg.
Complementary List	
heparin sodium	***Injection:*** *1000 IU/ml; 5000 IU/ml in 1-ml ampoule.*
protamine sulfate	***Injection:*** *10 mg/ml in 5-ml ampoule.*
□ *warfarin*	***Tablet:*** *0.5 mg; 1 mg; 2 mg; 5 mg (sodium salt).*

10.3 Other medicines for haemoglobinopathies

Complementary List	
*deferoxamine**	***Powder for injection:*** *500 mg (mesilate) in vial.* * *Deferasirox oral form may be an alternative, depending on cost and availability.*
hydroxycarbamide	***Solid oral dosage form:*** *200 mg; 500 mg; 1 g.*

11. BLOOD PRODUCTS AND PLASMA SUBSTITUTES

11.1 Plasma substitutes R

R The Committee requested a review to determine whether these medicines are essential for children.

11.2 Plasma fractions for specific use

All plasma fractions should comply with the WHO Requirements for the Collection, Processing and Quality Control of Blood, Blood Components and Plasma Derivatives (Revised 1992). (WHO Technical Report Series, No. 840, 1994, Annex 2).

Complementary List	
□ *factor VIII concentrate*	***Dried.***

11. BLOOD PRODUCTS AND PLASMA SUBSTITUTES *(continued)*

Medicine	Dosage form and strength
□ *factor IX complex (coagulation factors, II, VII, IX, X) concentrate*	***Dried.***
human normal immunoglobulin	***Intramuscular administration:*** *16% protein solution.** ***Intravenous administration:*** *5%; 10% protein solution.*** ***Subcutaneous administration:*** *15%; 16% protein solution.** ** Indicated for primary immune deficiency.* *** Indicated for primary immune deficiency and Kawasaki disease.*

12. CARDIOVASCULAR MEDICINES

~~12.1 Antianginal medicines~~

12.2 Antiarrhythmic medicines R

R The Committee noted the potential importance of these medicines and requested a review to determine which of these medicines are essential for children.

12.3 Antihypertensive medicines

Medicine	Dosage form and strength
□ enalapril	**Tablet:** 2.5 mg; 5 mg (as hydrogen maleate).

12.4 Medicines used in heart failure

Medicine	Dosage form and strength
digoxin	**Injection:** 250 micrograms/ml in 2-ml ampoule. **Oral liquid:** 50 micrograms/ml. **Tablet:** 62.5 micrograms; 250 micrograms.
furosemide	**Injection:** 10 mg/ml in 2-ml ampoule. **Oral liquid:** 20 mg/5 ml. **Tablet:** 40 mg.
Complementary List	
dopamine R	***Injection:*** *40 mg (hydrochloride) in 5-ml vial.* R Review of safety and efficacy of dopamine in children.

~~12.5 Antithrombotic medicines~~

12.6 Lipid-lowering agents R

R The Committee noted the potential importance of these medicines in children but requested a review of the section before endorsing any medicine as essential.

13. DERMATOLOGICAL MEDICINES (topical)

13.1 Antifungal medicines

□ miconazole	**Cream or ointment:** 2% (nitrate).
terbinafine	**Cream:** 1% **or Ointment:** 1% terbinafine hydrochloride.

13.2 Anti-infective medicines R

R The Committee requested a review of safety of topical antibiotics including tetracycline ointment in neonates.

mupirocin	**Cream (as mupirocin calcium):** 2%. **Ointment:** 2%.
potassium permanganate	**Aqueous solution:** 1:10 000.
silver sulfadiazine [a]	**Cream:** 1%. [a] >2 months.

13.3 Anti-inflammatory and antipruritic medicines

□ betamethasone [a]	**Cream or ointment:** 0.1% (as valerate). [a] Hydrocortisone preferred in neonates.
calamine	**Lotion.**
hydrocortisone	**Cream or ointment:** 1% (acetate).

13.4 Medicines affecting skin differentiation and proliferation

benzoyl peroxide	**Cream or lotion:** 5%.
coal tar	**Solution:** 5%.
□ podophyllum resin	**Solution:** 10% to 25%.
salicylic acid	**Solution:** 5%.
urea	**Cream or ointment:** 5%; 10%.

13.5 Scabicides and pediculicides

□ benzyl benzoate [a]	**Lotion:** 25%. [a] >2 years.
permethrin	**Cream:** 5%. **Lotion:** 1%.

14. DIAGNOSTIC AGENTS

14.1 Ophthalmic medicines

fluorescein	**Eye drops:** 1% (sodium salt).
□ tropicamide	**Eye drops:** 0.5%.

14.2 Radiocontrast media R

R The Committee requested a review of possible alternative contrast agents for use in children.

Complementary List

barium sulfate	***Aqueous suspension.***

15. DISINFECTANTS AND ANTISEPTICS

15.1 Antiseptics

□ chlorhexidine	**Solution:** 5% (digluconate); 20% (digluconate) (needs to be diluted prior to use for cord care).
□ ethanol	**Solution:** 70% (denatured).
□ polyvidone iodine	**Solution:** 10% (equivalent to 1% available iodine).

15.2 Disinfectants

□ chlorine base compound	**Powder:** (0.1% available chlorine) for solution.
□ chloroxylenol	**Solution:** 4.8%.
glutaral	**Solution:** 2%.

16. DIURETICS

furosemide	**Injection:** 10 mg/ml in 2-ml ampoule. **Oral liquid:** 20 mg/5 ml. **Tablet:** 10 mg; 20 mg; 40 mg.

Complementary List

□ *hydrochlorothiazide*	***Tablet (scored):*** *25 mg.*
mannitol	***Injectable solution:*** *10%; 20%.*
spironolactone	***Oral liquid:*** *5 mg/5 ml; 10 mg/5 ml; 25 mg/5 ml.* ***Tablet:*** *25 mg.*

17. GASTROINTESTINAL MEDICINES

Complementary List

□ *pancreatic enzymes*	*Age-appropriate formulations and doses including lipase, protease and amylase.*

17.1 Antiulcer medicines

□ omeprazole	**Powder for oral liquid:** 20 mg; 40 mg sachets. **Solid oral dosage form:** 10 mg; 20 mg; 40 mg.
□ ranitidine*	**Injection:** 25 mg/ml (as hydrochloride) in 2-ml ampoule. **Oral liquid:** 75 mg/5 ml (as hydrochloride). **Tablet:** 150 mg (as hydrochloride). * The Expert Committee has requested a review of the comparative effectiveness and safety, for possible deletion of this class of medicine at its next meeting.

17.2 Antiemetic medicines

dexamethasone	**Injection:** 4 mg/ml in 1-ml ampoule (as disodium phosphate salt). **Oral liquid:** 0.5 mg/5 ml; 2 mg/5 ml. **Solid oral dosage form:** 0.5 mg; 0.75 mg; 1.5 mg; 4 mg.
metoclopramide [a]	**Injection:** 5 mg (hydrochloride)/ml in 2-ml ampoule. **Oral liquid:** 5 mg/5 ml. **Tablet:** 10 mg (hydrochloride). [a] Not in neonates.
ondansetron [a]	**Injection:** 2 mg base/ml in 2-ml ampoule (as hydrochloride). **Oral liquid:** 4 mg base/ 5 ml. **Solid oral dosage form:** Eq 4 mg base; Eq 8 mg base. [a] >1 month.

~~17.3 Anti-inflammatory medicines~~

17.4 Laxatives [R]

[R] The Committee noted the potential importance of these medicines in children but requested a review of the section before endorsing any medicine as essential.

17. GASTROINTESTINAL MEDICINES *(continued)*

17.5 Medicines used in diarrhoea

17.5.1 *Oral rehydration*

oral rehydration salts	glucose:	75 mEq
	sodium:	75 mEq **or** mmol/L
	chloride:	65 mEq **or** mmol/L
	potassium:	20 mEq **or** mmol/L
	citrate:	10 mmol/L
	osmolarity:	245 mOsm/L
	glucose:	13.5 g/L
	sodium chloride:	2.6 g/L
	potassium chloride:	1.5 g/L
	trisodium citrate dihydrate+:	2.9 g/L

+ trisodium citrate dihydrate may be replaced by sodium hydrogen carbonate (sodium bicarbonate) 2.5 g/L. However, as the stability of this latter formulation is very poor under tropical conditions, it is only recommended when manufactured for immediate use.

Powder for dilution in 200 ml; 500 ml; 1 L.

17.5.2 *Medicines for diarrhoea in children*

zinc sulfate* — **Solid oral dosage form:** 20 mg.

* In acute diarrhoea zinc sulfate should be used as an adjunct to oral rehydration salts.

~~17.5.3 *Antidiarrhoeal (symptomatic) medicines in adults*~~

18. HORMONES, OTHER ENDOCRINE MEDICINES AND CONTRACEPTIVES

18.1 Adrenal hormones and synthetic substitutes

fludrocortisone	**Tablet:** 100 micrograms (acetate).
hydrocortisone	**Tablet:** 5 mg; 10 mg; 20 mg.

~~18.2 Androgens~~

~~18.3 Contraceptives~~

~~18.3.1 *Oral hormonal contraceptives*~~

~~18.3.2 *Injectable hormonal contraceptives*~~

~~18.3.3 *Intrauterine devices*~~

~~18.3.4 *Barrier methods*~~

18. HORMONES, OTHER ENDOCRINE MEDICINES AND CONTRACEPTIVES *(continued)*

~~18.3.5 *Implantable contraceptives*~~

~~18.4 Estrogens~~

18.5 Insulins and other medicines used for diabetes

glucagon	**Injection:** 1 mg/ml.
insulin injection (soluble)	**Injection:** 100 IU/ml in 10-ml vial.
intermediate-acting insulin	**Injection:** 100 IU/ml in 10-ml vial (as compound insulin zinc suspension **or** isophane insulin).
Complementary List	
metformin	***Tablet:*** *500 mg (hydrochloride).*

~~18.6 Ovulation inducers~~

~~18.7 Progestogens~~

18.8 Thyroid hormones and antithyroid medicines

levothyroxine	**Tablet:** 25 micrograms; 50 micrograms; 100 micrograms (sodium salt).
Complementary List	
Lugol's solution	***Oral liquid:*** *about 130 mg total iodine/ml.*
potassium iodide	***Tablet:*** *60 mg.*
propylthiouracil R	***Tablet:*** *50 mg.* R Review of use of propylthiouracil in children and appropriateness of carbimazole as an alternative.

19. IMMUNOLOGICALS

19.1 Diagnostic agents

All tuberculins should comply with the WHO Requirements for Tuberculins (Revised 1985). WHO Expert Committee on Biological Standardization. Thirty-sixth report (*WHO Technical Report Series*, No. 745, 1987, Annex 1).

tuberculin, purified protein derivative (PPD)	**Injection.**

19.2 Sera and immunoglobulins

All plasma fractions should comply with the WHO Requirements for the Collection, Processing and Quality Control of Blood, Blood Components and Plasma Derivatives (Revised 1992). WHO Expert Committee on Biological Standardization. Forty-third report (*WHO Technical Report Series*, No. 840, 1994, Annex 2).

19. IMMUNOLOGICALS *(continued)*

antitetanus immunoglobulin (human)	**Injection:** 500 IU in vial.
antivenom immunoglobulin*	**Injection.** * Exact type to be defined locally.
diphtheria antitoxin	**Injection:** 10 000 IU; 20 000 IU in vial.
□ rabies immunoglobulin	**Injection:** 150 IU/ml in vial.

19.3 Vaccines

Selection of vaccines from the Model List will need to be determined by each country after consideration of international recommendations, epidemiology and national priorities. The list below details the vaccines for which there is either a recommendation from the Strategic Advisory Group of Experts on Immunization (SAGE) (http://www.who.int/immunization/sage_conclusions/en/index.html) and/or a WHO position paper (http://www.who.int/immunization/documents/positionpapers/en/index.html). This site will be updated as new position papers are published and contains the most recent information and recommendations. All vaccines should comply with the WHO Requirements for Biological Substances.

The Committee noted the need for vaccines used in children to be polyvalent.

BCG vaccine

cholera vaccine

diphtheria vaccine

Haemophilus influenzae type b vaccine

hepatitis A vaccine

hepatitis B vaccine

influenza vaccine

Japanese encephalitis vaccine

measles vaccine

meningococcal meningitis vaccine

mumps vaccine

pertussis vaccine

pneumococcal vaccine

poliomyelitis vaccine

rabies vaccine

19. IMMUNOLOGICALS *(continued)*

rotavirus vaccine

rubella vaccine

tetanus vaccine

typhoid vaccine

varicella vaccine

yellow fever vaccine

20. MUSCLE RELAXANTS (PERIPHERALLY-ACTING) AND CHOLINESTERASE INHIBITORS R

R The Expert Committee has requested a review of this section at its next meeting.

neostigmine	**Injection:** 500 micrograms in 1-ml ampoule; 2.5 mg (metilsulfate) in 1-ml ampoule. **Tablet:** 15 mg (bromide).
suxamethonium	**Injection:** 50 mg (chloride)/ml in 2-ml ampoule. **Powder for injection:** (chloride), in vial.
□ vecuronium	**Powder for injection:** 10 mg (bromide) in vial.
Complementary List	
pyridostigmine	***Injection:*** *1 mg in 1-ml ampoule.* ***Tablet:*** *60 mg (bromide).*

21. OPHTHALMOLOGICAL PREPARATIONS R

R The Committee requested a review of newer medicines for potential additions to this list.

21.1 Anti-infective agents

aciclovir	**Ointment:** 3% W/W.
□ gentamicin	**Solution (eye drops):** 0.3% (sulfate).
□ tetracycline	**Eye ointment:** 1% (hydrochloride).

21.2 Anti-inflammatory agents

□ prednisolone	**Solution (eye drops):** 0.5% (sodium phosphate).

21.3 Local anaesthetics

□ tetracaine [a]	**Solution (eye drops):** 0.5% (hydrochloride). [a] Not in preterm neonates.

21. OPHTHALMOLOGICAL PREPARATIONS R *(continued)*

~~21.4 Miotics and antiglaucoma medicines~~

21.5 Mydriatics

atropine* [a]	**Solution (eye drops):** 0.1%; 0.5%; 1% (sulfate). * **Or** homatropine (hydrobromide) **or** cyclopentolate (hydrochloride). [a] >3 months.

Complementary List

epinephrine (adrenaline) R	***Solution (eye drops):*** *2% (as hydrochloride).* R Review of anti-infective eye drops, identifying which are most appropriate for use in children.

~~22. OXYTOCICS AND ANTIOXYTOCICS~~

~~22.1 Oxytocics~~

~~22.2 Antioxytocics (tocolytics)~~

23. PERITONEAL DIALYSIS SOLUTION

Complementary List

intraperitoneal dialysis solution (of appropriate composition)	***Parenteral solution.***

24. MEDICINES FOR MENTAL AND BEHAVIOURAL DISORDERS R

R The Committee noted the potential importance of these medicines in children for a variety of disorders and requests a review of the entire section.

24.1 Medicines used in psychotic disorders

Complementary List

chlorpromazine	***Injection:*** *25 mg (hydrochloride)/ml in 2-ml ampoule.* ***Oral liquid:*** *25 mg (hydrochloride)/5 ml.* ***Tablet:*** *10 mg; 25 mg; 50 mg; 100 mg (hydrochloride).*
haloperidol	***Injection:*** *5 mg in 1-ml ampoule.* ***Oral liquid:*** *2 mg/ml.* ***Solid oral dosage form:*** *0.5 mg; 2 mg; 5 mg.*

24. MEDICINES FOR MENTAL AND BEHAVIOURAL DISORDERS R *(continued)*

24.2 Medicines used in mood disorders

24.2.1 *Medicines used in depressive disorders*

Complementary List

fluoxetine [a]	***Solid oral dosage form:*** *20 mg (as hydrochloride).* [a] >8 years.

24.2.2 *Medicines used in bipolar disorders* R

24.3 Medicines for anxiety disorders R

24.4 Medicines used for obsessive compulsive disorders R

24.5 Medicines for disorders due to psychoactive substance use R

25. MEDICINES ACTING ON THE RESPIRATORY TRACT

25.1 Antiasthmatic medicines

□ budesonide	**Inhalation (aerosol):** 100 micrograms per dose; 200 micrograms per dose.
epinephrine (adrenaline)	**Injection:** 1 mg (as hydrochloride **or** hydrogen tartrate) in 1-ml ampoule.
□ salbutamol	**Injection:** 50 micrograms (as sulfate)/ml in 5-ml ampoule. **Metered dose inhaler (aerosol):** 100 micrograms (as sulfate) per dose. **Respirator solution for use in nebulizers:** 5 mg (as sulfate)/ml.

26. SOLUTIONS CORRECTING WATER, ELECTROLYTE AND ACID-BASE DISTURBANCES

26.1 Oral

oral rehydration salts	See section 17.5.1.
potassium chloride	**Powder for solution.**

26.2 Parenteral

glucose	**Injectable solution:** 5% (isotonic); 10% (hypertonic); 50% (hypertonic).
glucose with sodium chloride	**Injectable solution:** 5% glucose, 0.9% sodium chloride (equivalent to 150 mmol/L Na+ and 150 mmol/L Cl-); 5% glucose, 0.45% sodium chloride (equivalent to 75 mmol/L Na+ and 75 mmol/L Cl-).

26. SOLUTIONS CORRECTING WATER, ELECTROLYTE AND ACID-BASE DISTURBANCES *(continued)*	
potassium chloride	**Solution for dilution:** 7.5% (equivalent to K 1 mmol/ml and Cl 1 mmol/ml); 15% (equivalent to K 2 mmol/ml and Cl 2 mmol/ml).
sodium chloride	**Injectable solution:** 0.9% isotonic (equivalent to Na+ 154 mmol/L, Cl- 154 mmol/L).
sodium hydrogen carbonate	**Injectable solution:** 1.4% isotonic (equivalent to Na+ 167 mmol/L, HCO_3- 167 mmol/L). **Solution:** 8.4% in 10-ml ampoule (equivalent to Na+ 1000 mmol/L, HCO_3-1000 mmol/L).
□ sodium lactate, compound solution	**Injectable solution.**
26.3 Miscellaneous	
water for injection	2-ml; 5-ml; 10-ml ampoules.

27. VITAMINS AND MINERALS R

R The Committee noted the need for a review of this section of the list to meet public health needs in children.

ascorbic acid	**Tablet:** 50 mg.
cholecalciferol*	**Oral liquid:** 400 IU/ml. **Solid oral dosage form:** 400 IU; 1000 IU. * Ergocalciferol can be used as an alternative.
iodine	**Capsule:** 200 mg. **Iodized oil:** 1 ml (480 mg iodine); 0.5 ml (240 mg iodine) in ampoule (oral **or** injectable); 0.57 ml (308 mg iodine) in dispenser bottle.
pyridoxine	**Tablet:** 25 mg (hydrochloride).
retinol	**Capsule:** 100 000 IU; 200 000 IU (as palmitate). **Oral oily solution:** 100 000 IU (as palmitate)/ml in multidose dispenser. **Tablet (sugar-coated):** 10 000 IU (as palmitate). **Water-miscible injection:** 100 000 IU (as palmitate) in 2-ml ampoule.
riboflavin	**Tablet:** 5 mg.
sodium fluoride	In any appropriate topical formulation.

27. VITAMINS AND MINERALS R *(continued)*

thiamine	**Tablet:** 50 mg (hydrochloride).
Complementary List	
calcium gluconate	***Injection:*** *100 mg/ml in 10-ml ampoule.*

28. EAR, NOSE AND THROAT CONDITIONS IN CHILDREN R

R Review of role of leukotriene antagonists in the management of childhood allergic rhinitis.

acetic acid	**Topical:** 2%, in alcohol.
□ budesonide	**Nasal spray:** 100 micrograms per dose.
□ ciprofloxacin	**Topical:** 0.3% drops (as hydrochloride).
□ xylometazoline [a]	**Nasal spray:** 0.05%. [a] Not in children less than 3 months.

29. SPECIFIC MEDICINES FOR NEONATAL CARE

caffeine citrate	**Injection:** 20 mg/ml (equivalent to 10 mg caffeine base/ml). **Oral liquid:** 20 mg/ml (equivalent to 10 mg caffeine base/ml).
Complementary List	
□ *ibuprofen*	***Solution for injection:*** *5 mg/ml.*
□ *prostaglandin E*	***Solution for injection:*** ***Prostaglandin E1:*** *0.5 mg/ml in alcohol.* ***Prostaglandin E2:*** *1 mg/ml.*
surfactant	***Suspension for intratracheal instillation:*** *25 mg/ml **or** 80 mg/ml.*

Appendix

Essential medicines that can be used in neonates

CORE	
oxygen	**Inhalation** (medicinal gas) (*Section 1.1*)
lidocaine	**Injectable solution:** 1%; 2% (hydrochloride) in vial **Topical forms:** 2% to 4% (hydrochloride) (*Section 1.2*)
□ midazolam	**Injection:** 1 mg/ml. **Oral liquid:** 2 mg/ml (*Section 1.3*)
morphine	**Injection:** 10 mg (as morphine hydrochloride or morphine sulfate) in 1-ml ampoule (*Sections 1.3 and 2.2*) **Oral liquid:** 10 mg (as morphine hydrochloride or morphine sulfate)/5 ml (*Section 2.2*)
paracetamol	**Oral liquid:** 125 mg/5 ml **Suppository:** 60 mg (*Section 2.1*)
epinephrine	**Injection:** 1 mg (as hydrochloride or hydrogen tartrate) in 1-ml ampoule (*Sections 3 and 25.1*)
calcium gluconate	**Injection:** 100 mg/ml in 10-ml ampoule (*Section 4.2*)
naloxone	**Injection:** 400 micrograms (as hydrochloride) in 1-ml ampoule (*Section 4.2*)
phenobarbital	**Injection:** 200 mg/ml (phenobarbital sodium) (*Section 5*)
phenytoin	**Injection:** 50 mg/ml in 5-ml ampoule (as sodium salt) **Oral liquid suspension:** 25 mg to 30 mg/5 ml (*Section 5*)
amoxicillin as trihydrate (as sodium salt)	**Powder for oral liquid:** 125 mg (anhydrous)/5 ml; 250 mg (anhydrous)/5 ml (*Section 6.2.1*)
ampicillin	**Injection:** 500 mg (as sodium salt) in vial (*Section 6.2.1*)
benzylpenicillin (penicillin G)	**Powder for injection:** 600 mg (= 1 million IU); (sodium or potassium salt) in vial (*Section 6.2.1*)
cefotaxime	**Powder for reconstitution:** 500 mg (*Section 6.2.1*)

CORE *(continued)*	
ceftriaxone [a]	**Powder for reconstitution:** 250 mg (as sodium salt) in vial (*Section 6.2.1*) [a] Not in infants aged <41 weeks corrected gestational age.
cloxacillin	**Injection:** 500 mg (as sodium salt) in vial (*Section 6.2.1*)
procaine benzylpenicillin	**Suspension for intramuscular injection:** 1 g (*Section 6.2.1*)
□ erythromycin	**Powder for oral liquid:** 125 mg (as stearate or ethyl succinate) in 5 ml (*Section 6.2.2*)
gentamicin	**Injection:** 10 mg (as sulfate)/ml in 2-ml vial (*Section 6.2.2*) **Solution (eye drops):** 0.3% (as sulfate) (*Section 21.1*)
fluconazole	**Injection:** 2 mg/ml in vial **Oral liquid:** 50 mg/5 ml (*Section 6.3*)
nystatin	**Oral liquid:** 50 mg/5 ml or 100 000 IU/ml (*Section 6.3*)
zidovudine	**Oral liquid:** 50 mg/5 ml **Solution for injection:** 10 mg/ml (*Section 6.4.2.1*)
nevirapine	**Oral liquid:** 50 mg/5 ml (*Section 6.4.2.2*)
phytomenadione	**Injection:** 1 mg/ml in 5-ml ampoule (*Section 10.2*)
oral rehydration salts	glucose: 75 mEq sodium: 75 mEq or mmol/L chloride: 65 mEq or mmol/L potassium: 20 mEq or mmol/L citrate: 10 mmol/L osmolarity: 245 mOsm/L glucose: 13.5 g/L sodium chloride: 2.6 g/L potassium chloride: 1.5 g/L trisodium citrate dihydrate:* 2.9 g/L (*Sections 17.5.1 and 26.1*) * trisodium citrate dihydrate may be replaced by sodium hydrogen carbonate (sodium bicarbonate) 2.5 g/L. However, as the stability of this latter formulation is very poor under tropical conditions, it is only recommended when manufactured for immediate use.

CORE *(continued)*	
antitetanus immunoglobulin	500 IU vial (*Section 19.2*)
caffeine citrate	**Injection:** 20 mg/ml (equivalent to 10 mg caffeine base/ml) **Oral liquid:** 20 mg/ml (equivalent to 10 mg caffeine base/ml) (*Section 25.2*)
glucose	**Injectable solution:** 10% (*Section 26.2*)
potassium chloride	**Solution for injection:** 7.5% (equivalent to K 1 mmol/ml and Cl 1 mmol/ml) (*Section 26.2*)
sodium chloride	**Injectable solution:** 0.9% isotonic (equivalent to Na+ 154 mmol/L, Cl- 154 mmol/L) (*Section 26.2*)
water for injection	**Solution for injection:** 2-ml; 5-ml; 10-ml ampoules (*Section 26.3*)
cholecalciferol	**Oral liquid:** 400 IU/ml (*Section 27*)
COMPLEMENTARY	
atropine sulfate	**Injection:** 1 mg (as sulfate) in 1-ml ampoule (*Sections 1 and 4*)
hydrocortisone	**Powder for injection:** 100 mg (as sodium succinate) in vial (*Sections 3 and 8.3*)
imipenem + cilastatin	**Powder for injection:** 250 mg (as monohydrate) + 250 mg (as sodium salt) in vial (*Section 6.2.1*)
metronidazole	**Injection:** 500 mg in 100-ml vial (*Sections 6.2.2 and 6.5.1*)
vancomycin	**Powder for injection:** 250 mg (as hydrochloride) in vial (*Section 6.2.2*)
amikacin	**Solution for injection:** 50 mg/ml (*Section 6.2.4*)
aciclovir	**Solution for injection:** 250 mg/10 ml (*Section 6.4.1*)
amphotericin B	**Injection:** 50 mg in vial (*Section 6.5.2*)
digoxin	**Injection:** 100 micrograms/ml **Oral liquid:** 50 micrograms/ml (*Section 12.4*)
dopamine	**Injection:** 40 mg/ml as hydrochloride in 5-ml vial (*Section 12.4*)
ranitidine	**Injection:** 25 mg/ml in 2-ml ampoule (*Section 17.1*)
insulin	**Injection:** 100 IU/ml in 10-ml vial (*Section 18.5*)

Annex 3

The Anatomical Therapeutic Chemical (ATC) Classification System

The following list provides the corresponding Anatomical Therapeutic Chemical (ATC) classification codes for all items on the 17th WHO Model List of Essential Medicines and the 3rd WHO Model List of Essential Medicines for Children, sorted by ATC code number.

ATC code	ATC group/medicine or item	Section
A	ALIMENTARY TRACT AND METABOLISM	
A02B	**Drugs for peptic ulcer and gastro-oesophageal reflux disease (GORD)**	
A02BA	*H_2-receptor antagonists*	
A02BA02	ranitidine	17.1
A02BC	*Proton pump inhibitors*	
A02BC01	omeprazole	17.1
A03	**Drugs for functional gastrointestinal disorders**	
A03B	**Belladonna and derivatives, plain**	
A03BA	*Belladonna alkaloids, tertiary amines*	
A03BA01	atropine	1.3; 4.2
A03F	**Propulsives**	
A03FA	*Propulsives*	
A03FA01	metoclopramide	17.2
A04	**Antiemetics and antinauseants**	
A04A	**Antiemetics and antinauseants**	
A04AA	*Serotonin (5HT3) antagonists*	
A04AA01	ondansetron	17.2
A06	**Laxatives**	
A06A	**Laxatives**	
A06AB	*Contact laxatives*	
A06AB06	senna glycosides*	17.4
A07	**Antidiarrheals, intestinal antiinflammatory/antiinfective agents**	
A07A	**Intestinal antiinfectives**	
A07AA	*Antibiotics*	
A07AA06	paromomycin	6.5.2

ATC code	ATC group/medicine or item	Section
A07B	**Intestinal adsorbents**	
A07BA	*Charcoal preparations*	
A07BA01	medicinal charcoal*	4.1
A07C	**Electrolytes with carbohydrates**	
A07CA	*Oral rehydration salt formulations**	17.5.1; 26.1
A07E	**Intestinal antiinflammatory agents**	
A07EA	*Corticosteroids for local use*	
A07EA02	hydrocortisone	17.3
A07EC	*Aminosalicylic acid and similar agents*	
A07EC01	sulfasalazine	2.4; 17.3
A09	**Digestives, incl. enzymes**	
A09A	**Digestives, incl. enzymes**	
A09AA	*Enzyme preparations*	
A09AA02	multienzymes (lipase, protease, etc.)*	17
A10	**Drugs used in diabetes**	
A10A	**Insulins and analogues**	
A10AB	*Insulins and analogues for injection, fast-acting*	
A10AB	insulin injection (soluble)*	18.5
A10AC	*Insulins and analogues for injection, intermediate-acting*	
A10AC	insulin, intermediate-acting*	18.5
A10B	**Blood glucose lowering drugs, excl. insulins**	
A10BA	*Biguanides*	
A10BA02	metformin	18.5
A10BB	*Sulfonamides, urea derivatives*	
A10BB01	glibenclamide	18.5
A11	**Vitamins**	
A11C	**Vitamin A and D, incl. combinations of the two**	
A11CA	*Vitamin A, plain*	
A11CA01	retinol	27
A11CC	*Vitamin D and analogues*	
A11CC01	ergocalciferol	27
A11CC05	colecalciferol*	27
A11D	**Vitamin B_1, plain and in combination with vitamin B_6 and B_{12}**	
A11DA	*Vitamin B1, plain*	
A11DA01	thiamine	27

ATC code	ATC group/medicine or item	Section
A11G	**Ascorbic acid (vitamin C), incl. combinations**	
A11GA	*Ascorbic acid (vitamin C), plain*	
A11GA01	ascorbic acid	27
A11H	**Other plain vitamin preparations**	
A11HA	*Other plain vitamin preparations*	
A11HA01	nicotinamide	27
A11HA02	pyridoxine	27
A11HA04	riboflavin	27
A12	**Mineral supplements**	
A12A	**Calcium**	
A12AA	*Calcium*	
A12AA03	calcium gluconate	4.2; 27
A12C	**Other mineral supplements**	
A12CB	*Zinc*	
A12CB01	zinc sulfate	17.5.2
A12CD	*Fluoride*	
A12CD01	sodium fluoride	27
A12CX	*Other mineral products**	27
B	**BLOOD AND BLOOD FORMING ORGANS**	
B01	**Antithrombotic agents**	
B01A	**Antithrombotic agents**	
B01AA	*Vitamin K antagonists*	
B01AA03	warfarin	10.2
B01AB	*Heparin group*	
B01AB01	heparin*	10.2
B01AC	*Platelet aggregation inhibitors excl. heparin*	
B01AC06	acetylsalicylic acid	12.5
B01AD	*Enzymes*	
B01AD01	streptokinase	12.5
B02	**Antihemorrhagics**	
B02A	**Antifibrinolytics**	
B02AA	*Amino acids*	
B02AA02	tranexamic acid	10.2
B02B	**Vitamin K and other hemostatics**	
B02BA	*Vitamin K*	
B02BA01	phytomenadione	10.2

ATC code	ATC group/medicine or item	Section
B02BD	*Blood coagulation factors*	
B02BD01	coagulation factor IX, II, VII and X in combination*	11.2
B02BD02	coagulation factor VIII*	11.2
B03	**Antianemic preparations**	
B03A	**Iron preparations***	10.1
B03AD	*Iron in combination with folic acid**	10.1
B03B	**Vitamin B_{12} and folic acid**	
B03BA	*Vitamin B_{12} (cyanocobalamin and analogues)*	
B03BA03	hydroxocobalamin	10.1
B03BB	*Folic acid and derivatives*	
B03BB01	folic acid	10.1
B05	**Blood substitutes and perfusion solutions**	
B05A	**Blood and related products**	
B05AA	*Blood substitutes and plasma protein fractions*	
B05AA05	dextran*	11.1
B05B	**I.V. solutions**	
B05BA	*Solutions for parenteral nutrition*	
B05BA03	carbohydrates*	26.2
B05BB	*Solutions affecting the electrolyte balance*	
B05BB01	electrolytes*	26.2
B05BB02	electrolytes with carbohydrates*	26.2
B05BC	*Solutions producing osmotic diuresis*	
B05BC01	mannitol	16
B05D	**Peritoneal dialytics**	
B05DA	*Isotonic solutions**	23
B05X	**I.V. solution additives**	
B05XA	*Electrolyte solutions*	
B05XA01	potassium chloride	26.1; 26.2
B05XA02	sodium bicarbonate*	26.2
B05XA03	sodium chloride	26.2
B05XA05	magnesium sulfate	5
C	**CARDIOVASCULAR SYSTEM**	
C01	**Cardiac therapy**	
C01A	**Cardiac glycosides**	
C01AA	*Digitalis glycosides*	
C01AA01	simvastatin	12.6
C01AA05	digoxin	12.2; 12.4

ATC code	ATC group/medicine or item	Section
C01B	**Antiarrhythmics, class I and III**	
C01BB	*Antiarrhythmics, class Ib*	
C01BB01	lidocaine	12.2
C01BD	*Antiarrhythmics, class III*	
C01BD01	amiodarone	12.2
C01C	**Cardiac stimulants excl. cardiac glycosides**	
C01CA	*Adrenergic and dopaminergic agents*	
C01CA04	dopamine	12.4
C01CA24	epinephrine (adrenaline)	3; 12.2; 25.1
C01D	**Vasodilators used in cardiac diseases**	
C01DA	*Organic nitrates*	
C01DA02	glyceryl trinitrate	12.1
C01DA08	isosorbide dinitrate	12.1
C01E	**Other cardiac preparations**	
C01EA	*Prostaglandins*	
C01EA01	alprostadil*	29
C02	**Antihypertensives**	
C02A	***Antiadrenergic agents, centrally acting***	
C02AB	*Methyldopa*	
C02AB01	methyldopa (levorotatory)*	12.3
C02D	**Arteriolar smooth muscle, agents acting on**	
C02DB	*Hydrazinophthalazine derivatives*	
C02DB02	hydrazaline	12.3
C02DD	*Nitroferricyanide derivatives*	
C02DD01	nitroprusside*	12.3
C03	**Diuretics**	
C03A	**Low-ceiling diuretics, thiazides**	
C03AA	*Thiazides, plain*	
C03AA03	hydrochlorothiazide	12.3; 12.4; 16
C03C	**High-ceiling diuretics**	
C03CA	*Sulfonamides, plain*	
C03CA01	furosemide	12.4; 16
C03D	**Potassium-sparing agents**	
C03DA	*Aldosterone antagonists*	
C03DA01	spironolactone	16
C03DB	*Other potassium-sparing agents*	
C03DB01	amiloride	16

ATC code	ATC group/medicine or item	Section
C07	**Beta blocking agents**	
C07A	**Beta blocking agents**	
C07AA	*Beta blocking agents, non-selective*	
C07AA05	propranolol	7.2
C07AB	*Beta blocking agents, selective*	
C07AB07	bisoprolol	12.1; 12.2; 12.3; 12.4
C08	**Calcium channel blockers**	
C08C	**Selective calcium channel blockers with mainly vascular effects**	
C08CA	*Dihydropyridine derivatives*	
C08CA01	amlodipine	12.3
C08CA05	nifedipine	22.2
C08D	**Selective calcium channel blockers with direct cardiac effects**	
C08DA	*Phenylalkylamine derivatives*	
C08DA01	verapamil	12.1; 12.2
C09	**Agents acting on the renin-angiotensin system**	
C09A	**ACE inhibitors, plain**	
C09AA	*ACE inhibitors, plain*	
C09AA02	enalapril	12.3; 12.4
D	**DERMATOLOGICALS**	
D01	**Antifungals for dermatological use**	
D01A	**Antifungals for topical use**	
D01AA	*Antibiotics*	
D01AA01	nystatin	6.3
D01AC	*Imidazole and triazole derivatives*	
D01AC02	miconazole	13.1
D01AE	*Other antifungals for topical use*	
D01AE12	salicylic acid	13.5
D01AE13	selenium sulfide	13.1
D01B	**Antifungals for systemic use**	
D01BA	*Antifungals for systemic use*	
D01BA01	griseofulvin	6.3
D01BA02	terbinafine	13.1
D02	**Emollients and protectives**	
D02A	*Emollients and protectives*	
D02AB	*Zinc products**	13.3

ATC code	ATC group/medicine or item	Section
D02AE	*Carbamide products*	
D02AE01	carbamide*	13.5
D05	**Antipsoriatics**	
D05A	**Antipsoriatics for topical use**	
D05AA	*Tars**	13.5
D05AC	*Antracen derivatives*	
D05AC01	dithranol	13.5
D06	**Antibiotics and chemotherapeutics for dermatological use**	
D06A	**Antibiotics for topical use**	
D06AX	*Other antibiotics for topical use*	
D06AX09	mupirocin	13.2
D06B	**Chemotherapeutics for topical use**	
D06BA	*Sulfonamides*	
D06BA01	silver sulfadiazine	13.2
D06BB	*Antivirals*	
D06BB04	podophyllotoxin*	13.5
D07	**Corticosteroids, dermatological preparations**	
D07A	**Corticosteroids, plain**	
D07AA	*Corticosteroids, weak (group I)*	
D07AA02	hydrocortisone	13.3
D07AC	*Corticosteroids, potent (group III)*	
D07AC01	betamethasone	13.3
D08	**Antiseptics and disinfectants**	
D08A	**Antiseptics and disinfectants**	
D08AC	*Biguanides and amidines*	
D08AC02	chlorhexidine	15.1
D08AE	*Phenol and derivatives*	
D08AE05	chloroxylenol	15.2
D08AG	*Iodine products*	
D08AG02	povidone-iodine*	15.1
D08AX	*Other antiseptics and disinfectants**	15.2
D08AX06	potassium permanganate	13.2
D08AX08	ethanol	15.1

ATC code	ATC group/medicine or item	Section
D10	**Anti-acne preparations**	
D10A	**Anti-acne preparations for topical use**	
D10AE	*Peroxides*	
D10AE01	benzoyl peroxide	13.5
G	**GENITO URINARY SYSTEM AND SEX HORMONES**	
G01	**Gynecological antiinfectives and antiseptics**	
G01A	**Antiinfectives and antiseptics, excl. combinations with corticosteroids**	
G01AF	*Imidazole derivatives*	
G01AF02	clotrimazole	6.3
G02	**Other gynecologicals**	
G02A	**Oxytocics**	
G02AB	*Ergot alkaloids*	
G02AB03	ergometrine	22.1
G02AD	*Prostaglandins*	
G02AD06	misoprostol	22.1
G02B	**Contraceptives for topical use**	
G02BA	*Intrauterine contraceptives*	
G02BA02	plastic IUD with copper*	18.3.3
G02BA03	plastic IUD with progesteron*	18.3.5
G02BB	*Intravaginal contraceptives**	18.3.4
G03	**Sex hormones and modulators of the genital system**	
G03A	**Hormonal contraceptives for systemic use**	
G03AA	*Progestogens and estrogens, fixed combinations*	
G03AA05	norethisterone and estrogen*	18.3.1
G03AA08	medroxyprogesterone and estrogen*	18.3.2
G03AB	*Progestogens and estrogens, sequential preparations*	
G03AB03	levonorgestrel and estrogen*	18.3.1
G03AC	*Progestogens*	
G03AC01	norethisterone*	18.3.2
G03AC03	levonorgestrel	18.3.1
G03AC06	medroxyprogesterone*	18.3.2; 18.7
G03B	**Androgens**	
G03BA	*3-oxoandrosten (4) derivatives*	
G03BA03	testosterone	18.2

ATC code	ATC group/medicine or item	Section
G03G	**Gonadotropins and other ovulation stimulants**	
G03GB	*Ovulation stimulants, synthetic*	
G03GB02	clomifene	18.6
G03X	**Other sex hormones and modulators of the genital system**	
G03XB	*Antiprogesterons*	
G03XB01	mifepristone	22.1
H	**SYSTEMIC HORMONAL PREPARATIONS, EXCL. SEX HORMONES AND INSULINS**	
H01	**Pituitary, hypothalamic hormones and analogues**	
H01B	**Posterior pituitary lobe hormones**	
H01BB	*Oxytocin and analogues*	
H01BB02	oxytocin	22.1
H02	**Corticosteroids for systemic use**	
H02A	**Corticosteroids for systemic use, plain**	
H02AA	*Mineralocorticoids*	
H02AA02	fludrocortisone	18.1
H02AB	*Glucocorticoids*	
H02AB02	dexamethasone	3; 8.3; 17.2
H02AB06	prednisolone	3; 8.3
H02AB09	hydrocortisone	3; 8.3
H03	**Thyroid therapy**	
H03A	**Thyroid preparations**	
H03AA	*Thyroid hormones*	
H03AA01	levothyroxine sodium*	18.8
H03B	**Antithyroid preparations**	
H03BA	*Thiouracils*	
H03BA02	propylthiouracil	18.8
H03C	**Iodine therapy**	
H03CA	*Iodine therapy**	18.8
H04	**Pancreatic hormones**	
H04A	**Glycogenolytic hormones**	
H04AA	*Glycogenolytic hormones*	
H04AA01	glucagon	18.5

ATC code	ATC group/medicine or item	Section
J	**ANTIINFECTIVES FOR SYSTEMIC USE**	
J01	**Antibacterials for systemic use**	
J01A	**Tetracyclines**	
J01AA	*Tetracyclines*	
J01AA02	doxycycline	6.2.2; 6.5.3.1; 6.5.3.2
J01B	**Amphenicols**	
J01BA	*Amphenicols*	
J01BA01	chloramphenicol	6.2.2
J01C	**Beta-lactam antibacterials, penicillins**	
J01CA	*Penicillins with extended spectrum*	
J01CA01	ampicillin	6.2.1
J01CA04	amoxicillin	6.2.1
J01CE	*Beta-lactamase sensitive penicillins*	
J01CE01	benzylpenicillin	6.2.1
J01CE02	phenoxymethylpenicillin	6.2.1
J01CE08	benzathine benzylpenicillin	6.2.1
J01CE09	procaine benzylpenicillin	6.2.1
J01CF	*Beta-lactamase resistant penicillins*	
J01CF02	cloxacillin	6.2.1
J01CR	*Combinations of penicillins, incl. beta-lactamase inhibitors*	
J01CR02	amoxicillin and enzyme inhibitor*	6.2.1
J01D	**Other beta-lactam antibacterials**	
J01DB	*First-generation cephalosporins*	
J01DB01	cefalexin	6.2.1
J01DB04	cefazolin	6.2.1
J01DD	*Third-generation cephalosporins*	
J01DD01	cefotaxime	6.2.1
J01DD02	ceftazidime	6.2.1
J01DD04	ceftriaxone	6.2.1
J01DD08	cefixime	6.2.1
J01DH	*Carbapenems*	
J01DH5	imipenem and enzyme inhibitor*	6.2.1
J01E	**Sulfonamides and trimethoprim**	
J01EA	*Trimethoprim and derivatives*	
J01EA01	trimethoprim	6.2.2

ATC code	ATC group/medicine or item	Section
J01EC	*Intermediate-acting sulfonamides*	
J01EC02	sulfadiazine	6.5.4
J01EE	*Combinations of sulfonamides and trimethoprim, incl. derivatives*	
J01EE01	sulfamethoxazole + trimethoprim	6.2.2; 6.5.4
J01F	**Macrolides, lincosamides and streptogramins**	
J01FA	*Macrolides*	
J01FA01	erythromycin	6.2.2
J01FA09	clarithromycin	6.2.2
J01FA10	azithromycin	6.2.2
J01FF	*Lincosamides*	
J01FF01	clindamycin	6.2.2
J01G	**Aminoglycoside antibacterials**	
J01GA	*Streptomycins*	
J01GA01	streptomycin	6.2.4
J01GB	*Other aminoglycosides*	
J01GB03	gentamicin	6.2.2
J01GB04	kanamycin	6.2.4
J01GB06	amikacin	6.2.4
J01M	**Quinolone antibacterials**	
J01MA	*Fluoroquinolones*	
J01MA01	ofloxacin	6.2.4
J01MA02	ciprofloxacin	6.2.2
J01X	**Other antibacterials**	
J01XA	*Glycopeptide antibacterials*	
J01XA01	vancomycin	6.2.2
J01XD	*Imidazole derivatives*	
J01XD01	metronidazole	6.2.2
J01XE	*Nitrofuran derivatives*	
J01XE01	nitrofurantoin	6.2.2
J01XX	*Other antibacterials*	
J01XX04	spectinomycin	6.2.2
J02	**Antimycotics for systemic use**	
J02A	**Antimycotics for systemic use**	
J02AA	*Antibiotics*	
J02AA01	amphotericin B	6.3; 6.5.2

ATC code	ATC group/medicine or item	Section
J02AC	*Triazole derivatives*	
J02AC01	fluconazole	6.3
J02AX	*Other antimycotics for systemic use*	
J02AX01	flucytosine	6.3
J04	**Antimycobacterials**	
J04A	**Drugs for treatment of tuberculosis**	
J04AA	*Aminosalicylic acid and derivatives*	
J04AA01	p-aminosalicylic acid*	6.2.4
J04AB	*Antibiotics*	
J04AB01	cycloserine	6.2.4
J04AB02	rifampicin	6.2.3; 6.2.4
J04AB04	rifabutin	6.2.4
J04AB30	capreomycin	6.2.4
J04AC	*Hydrazides*	
J04AC01	isoniazid	6.2.4
J04AD	*Thiocarbamide derivatives*	
J04AD03	ethionamide	6.2.4
J04AK	*Other drugs for treatment of tuberculosis*	
J04AK01	pyrazinamide	6.2.4
J04AK02	ethambutol	6.2.4
J04AM	*Combinations of drugs for treatment of tuberculosis**	6.2.4
J04AM02	rifampicin and isoniazid*	6.2.4
J04AM03	ethambutol and isoniazid*	6.2.4
J04AM05	rifampicin, pyrazinamide and isoniazid*	6.2.4
J04AM06	rifampicin, pyrazinamide, ethambutol and isoniazid*	6.2.4
J04B	**Drugs for treatment of lepra**	
J04BA	*Drugs for treatment of lepra*	
J04BA01	clofazimine	6.2.3
J04BA02	dapsone	6.2.3
J05	**Antivirals for systemic use**	
J05A	**Direct acting antivirals**	
J05AB	*Nucleosides and nucleotides excl. reverse transcriptase inhibitors*	
J05AB01	aciclovir	6.4.1
J05AB04	ribavirin	6.4.3
J05AE	*Protease inhibitors*	
J05AE01	saquinavir (SQV)	6.4.2.3

ATC code	ATC group/medicine or item	Section
J05AE02	indinavir (IDV)	6.4.2.3
J05AE03	ritonavir (r)	6.4.2.3
J05AE08	atazanavir	6.4.2.3
J05AE30	lopinavir + ritonavir (LPV/r)*	6.4.2.3
J05AF	*Nucleoside and nucleotide reverse transcriptase inhibitors*	
J05AF01	zidovudine (ZDV or AZT)	6.4.2.1
J05AF02	didanosine (ddI)	6.4.2.1
J05AF04	stavudine (d4T)	6.4.2.1
J05AF05	lamivudine (3TC)	6.4.2.1
J05AF06	abacavir (ABC)	6.4.2.1
J05AF07	tenofovir disoproxil fumarate	6.4.2.1
J05AF09	emtricitabine	6.4.2.1
J05AG	*Non-nucleoside reverse transcriptase inhibitors*	
J05AG01	nevirapine (NVP)	6.4.2.2
J05AG03	efavirenz (EFV or EFZ)	6.4.2.2
J05AR	*Antivirals for treatment of HIV infections, combinations*	
J05AR01	lamivudine + zidovudine (ZDV or AZT)	6.4.2
J05AR03	emtricitabine + tenofovir	6.4.2
J05AR05	lamivudine + nevirapine + zidovudine	6.4.2
J05AR06	efavirenz + emtricitabine + tenofovir	6.4.2
J05AR07	lamivudine + nevirapine + stavudine	6.4.2
J06	**Immune sera and immunoglobulins**	
J06A	**Immune sera**	
J06AA	*Immune sera*	
J06AA01	diphtheria antitoxin	19.2
J06AA03	snake venom antiserum*	19.2
J06B	**Immunoglobulins**	
J06BA	*Immunoglobulins, normal human*	
J06BA01	immunoglobulins, normal human, for extravascular admin*	11.2
J06BA02	immunoglobulins, normal human, for intravascular admin*	11.2
J06BB	*Specific immunoglobulins*	
J06BB01	anti-D immunoglobulin (human)	19.2
J06BB02	antitetanus immunoglobulin (human)	19.2
J06BB05	rabies immunoglobulin	19.2

ATC code	ATC group/medicine or item	Section
J07	**Vaccines**	
J07A	**Bacterial vaccines**	
J07AE	*Cholera vaccines*	19.3
J07AF	*Diphtheria vaccines*	
J07AF01	diphtheria toxoid*	19.3
J07AH	*Meningococcal vaccines**	19.3
J07AJ	*Pertussis vaccines*	
J07AJ01	pertussis vaccine	19.3
J07AL	*Pneumococcal vaccines*	
J07AL01	pneumococcus, purified polysaccharides antigen*	19.3
J07AM	*Tetanus vaccines*	
J07AM01	tetanus toxoid*	19.3
J07AN	*Tuberculosis vaccines*	
J07AN01	tuberculosis, live attenuated*	19.3
J07AP	*Typhoid vaccines*	
J07AP	typhoid vaccine	19.3
J07B	**Viral vaccines**	
J07BA	*Encephalitis vaccines*	
J07BA02	encephalitis, Japanese, inactivated, whole virus	19.3
J07BB	*Influenza vaccines*	
J07BB	influenza vaccine	19.3
J07BC	*Hepatitis vaccines*	
J07BC01	hepatitis B vaccine	19.3
J07BC02	hepatitis A vaccine	19.3
J07BD	*Measles vaccine**	
J07BD01	measles, live attenuated*	19.3
J07BE	*Mumps vaccines*	
J07BE01	mumps, live attenuated*	19.3
J07BF	*Poliomyelitis vaccine*	19.3
J07BG	*Rabies vaccine*	19.3
J07BH	*Rota virus diarrhea vaccines**	19.3
J07BJ	*Rubella vaccines*	19.3
J07BK	*Varicella zoster vaccines**	19.3

ATC code	ATC group/medicine or item	Section
J07BL	*Yellow fever vaccines*	19.3
J07C	**Bacterial and viral vaccines, combined**	
J07CA	*Bacterial and viral vaccines, combined**	19.3
L	**ANTINEOPLASTIC AND IMMUNOMODULATING AGENTS**	
L01	**Antineoplastic agents**	
L01A	**Alkylating agents**	
L01AA	*Nitrogen mustard analogues*	
L01AA01	cyclophosphamide	8.2
L01AA02	chlorambucil	8.2
L01AA06	ifosfamide	8.2
L01AX	*Other alkylating agents*	
L01AX04	dacarbazine	8.2
L01B	**Antimetabolites**	
L01BA	*Folic acid analogues*	
L01BA01	methotrexate	2.4; 8.2
L01BB	*Purine analogues*	
L01BB02	mercaptopurine	8.2
L01BC	*Pyrimidine analogues*	
L01BC01	cytarabine	8.2
L01BC02	fluorouracil	8.2; 13.5
L01C	**Plant alkaloids and other natural products**	
L01CA	*Vinca alkaloids and analogues*	
L01CA01	vinblastine	8.2
L01CA02	vincristine	8.2
L01CB	*Podophyllotoxin derivatives*	
L01CB01	etoposide	8.2
L01CD	*Taxanes*	
L01CD01	paclitaxel	8.2
L01CD02	docetaxel	8.2
L01D	**Cytotoxic antibiotics and related substances**	
L01DA	*Actinomycines*	
L01DA01	dactinomycin	8.2
L01DB	*Anthracyclines and related substances*	
L01DB01	doxorubicin	8.2
L01DB02	daunorubicin	8.2

ATC code	ATC group/medicine or item	Section
L01DC	*Other cytotoxic antibiotics*	
L01DC01	bleomycin	8.2
L01X	**Other antineoplastic agents**	
L01XA	Platinum compounds	
L01XA02	carboplatin	8.2
L01XB	*Methylhydrazines*	
L01XB01	procarbazine	8.2
L01XX	*Other antineoplastic agents*	
L01XX02	asparaginase	8.2
L01XX05	hydroxycarbamide	8.2; 10.3
L01XX09	miltefosine	6.5.2
L02	**Endocrine therapy**	
L02B	**Hormone antagonists and related agents**	
L02BA	*Anti-estrogens*	
L02BA01	tamoxifen	8.3
L04	**Immunosuppressants**	
L04A	**Immunosuppressants**	
L04AD	*Calcineurin inhibitors*	
L04AD01	ciclosporin	8.1
L04AX	*Other immunosuppressants*	
L04AX01	azathioprine	2.4; 8.1
M	**MUSCULO-SKELETAL SYSTEM**	
M01	**Antiinflammatory and antirheumatic products**	
M01A	**Antiinflammatory and antirheumatic products, non-steroids**	
M01AE	*Propionic acid derivatives*	
M01AE01	ibuprofen	2.1; 29
M01C	**Specific antirheumatic agents**	
M01CC	*Penicillamine and similar agents*	
M01CC01	penicillamine	2.4; 4.2
M03	**Muscle relaxants**	
M03A	**Muscle relaxants, peripherally acting agents**	
M03AA	*Curare alkaloids*	
M03AA01	alcuronium	20
M03AB	*Choline derivatives*	
M03AB01	suxamethonium	20

ATC code	ATC group/medicine or item	Section
M03AC	*Other quaternary ammonium compounds*	
M03AC03	vecuronium	20
M03AC04	atracurium	20
M04	**Antigout preparations**	
M04A	**Antigout preparations**	
M04AA	*Preparations inhibiting uric acid production*	
M04AA01	allopurinol	2.3
N	NERVOUS SYSTEM	
N01	**Anesthetics**	
N01A	**Anesthetics, general**	
N01AB	*Halogenated hydrocarbons*	
N01AB01	halothane	1.1.1
N01AB06	isoflurane	1.1.1
N01AX	*Other general anesthetics*	
N01AX03	ketamine	1.1.2
N01AX10	propofol	1.1.2
N01AX13	nitrous oxide	1.1.1
N01B	**Anesthetics, local**	
N01BB	*Amides*	
N01BB01	bupivacaine	1.2
N01BB02	lidocaine	1.2
N01BB52	lidocaine, combinations*	1.2
N02	**Analgesics**	
N02A	**Opioids**	
N02AA	*Natural opium alkaloids*	
N02AA01	morphine	1.3; 2.2
N02B	*Other analgesics and antipyretics*	
N02BA	*Salicylic acid and derivatives*	
N02BA01	acetylsalicylic acid	2.1; 7.1
N02BE	*Anilides*	
N02BE01	paracetamol	2.1; 7.1
N03	**Antiepileptics**	
N03A	**Antiepileptics**	
N03AA	*Barbiturates and derivatives*	
N03AA02	phenobarbital	5
N03AB	*Hydantoin derivatives*	
N03AB02	phenytoin	5

ATC code	ATC group/medicine or item	Section
N03AD	*Succinimide derivatives*	
N03AD01	ethosuximide	5
N03AF	*Carboxamide derivatives*	
N03AF01	carbamazepine	5; 24.2.2
N03AG	*Fatty acid derivatives*	
N03AG01	valproic acid	5; 24.2.2
N04	**Anti-parkinson drugs**	
N04A	**Anticholinergic agents**	
N04AA	*Tertiary amines*	
N04AA02	biperiden	9
N04B	**Dopaminergic agents**	
N04BA	*Dopa and dopa derivatives*	
N04BA02	levodopa and decarboxylase inhibitor*	9
N05	**Psycholeptics**	
N05A	**Antipsychotics**	
N05AA	*Phenothiazines with aliphatic side-chain*	
N05AA01	chlorpromazine	24.1
N05AB	*Phenothiazines with piperazine structure*	
N05AB02	fluphenazine	24.1
N05AD	*Butyrophenone derivatives*	
N05AD01	haloperidol	24.1
N05AN	*Lithium*	
N05AN01	lithium*	24.2.2
N05B	**Anxiolytics**	
N05BA	*Benzodiazepine derivatives*	
N05BA01	diazepam	5; 24.3
N05BA06	lorazepam	5
N05C	**Hypnotics and sedatives**	
N05CD	*Benzodiazepine derivatives*	
N05CD08	midazolam	1.3
N06	**Psychoanaleptics**	
N06A	**Antidepressants**	
N06AA	*Non-selective monoamine reuptake inhibitors*	
N06AA04	clomipramine	24.4
N06AA09	amitriptyline	24.2.1

ATC code	ATC group/medicine or item	Section
N06AB	*Selective serotonin reuptake inhibitors*	
N06AB03	fluoxetine	24.2.1
N06B	**Psychostimulants, agents used for ADHD and nootropics**	
N06BC	*Xanthine derivatives*	
N06BC01	caffeine citrate	29
N07	**Other nervous system drugs**	
N07A	**Parasympathomimetics**	
N07AA	*Anticholinesterases*	
N07AA01	neostigmine	20
N07AA02	pyridostigmine	20
N07B	**Drugs used in addictive disorders**	
N07BA	*Drugs used in nicotine dependence*	
N07BA01	nicotine replacement therapy*	24.5
N07BC	*Drugs used in opioid dependence*	
N07BC02	methadone	24.5
P	**ANTIPARASITIC PRODUCTS, INSECTICIDES AND REPELLENTS**	
P01	**Antiprotozoals**	
P01A	**Agents against amoebiasis and other protozoal diseases**	
P01AB	*Nitroimidazole derivatives*	
P01AB01	metronidazole	6.5.1
P01AC	*Dichloroacetamide derivatives*	
P01AC01	diloxanide	6.5.1
P01B	**Antimalarials**	
P01BA	*Aminoquinolines*	
P01BA01	chloroquine	2.4; 6.5.3.1; 6.5.3.2
P01BA03	primaquine	6.5.3.1
P01BA06	amodiaquine	6.5.3.1
P01BB	*Biguanides*	
P01BB01	proguanil	6.5.3.2
P01BC	*Methanolquinolines*	
P01BC01	quinine	6.5.3.1
P01BC02	mefloquine	6.5.3.1; 6.5.3.2

ATC code	ATC group/medicine or item	Section
P01BD	*Diaminopyrimidines*	
P01BD01	pyrimethamine	6.5.4
P01BD51	pyrimethamine, combinations*	6.5.3.1
P01BE	*Artemisinin and derivatives*	
P01BE02	artemether	6.5.3.1
P01BE03	artesunate	6.5.3.1
P01BE52	artemether, combinations*	6.5.3.1
P01C	**Agents against leishmaniasis and trypanosomiasis**	
P01CA	*Nitroimidazole derivatives*	
P01CA02	benznidazole	6.5.5.2
P01CB	*Antimony compounds*	
P01CB01	meglumine antimoniate	6.5.2
P01CB02	sodium stibogluconate	6.5.2
P01CC	*Nitrofuran derivatives*	
P01CC01	nifurtimox	6.5.5.1; 6.5.5.2
P01CD	*Arsenic compounds*	
P01CD01	melarsoprol	6.5.5.1
P01CX	*Other agents against leishmaniasis and trypanosomiasis*	
P01CX01	pentamidine isethionate*	6.5.4; 6.5.5.1
P01CX02	suramin sodium	6.5.5.1
P01CX03	eflornithine	6.5.5.1
P02	**Anthelmintics**	
P02B	**Antitrematodals**	
P02BA	*Quinoline derivatives and related substances*	
P02BA01	praziquantel	6.1.1; 6.1.3
P02BA02	oxamniquine	6.1.3
P02BX	*Other antitrematodal agents*	
P02BX04	triclabendazole	6.1.3
P02C	**Antinematodal agents**	
P02CA	*Benzimidazole derivatives*	
P02CA01	mebendazole	6.1.1
P02CA03	albendazole	6.1.1; 6.1.2
P02CB	*Piperazine and derivatives*	
P02CB02	diethylcarbamazine	6.1.2

ATC code	ATC group/medicine or item	Section
P02CC	*Tetrahydropyrimidine derivatives*	
P02CC01	pyrantel	6.1.1
P02CE	*Imidazothiazole derivatives*	
P02CE01	levamisole	6.1.1
P02CF	*Avermectines*	
P02CF01	ivermectin	6.1.2
P02D	**Anticestodals**	
P02DA	*Salicylic acid derivatives*	
P02DA01	niclosamide	6.1.1
P03	**Ectoparasiticides, incl. scabicides, insecticides and repellents**	
P03A	**Ectoparasiticides, incl. scabicides**	
P03AC	*Pyrethrines, incl. synthetic compounds*	
P03AC04	permethrin	13.6
P03AX	*Other ectoparasiticides, incl. scabicides*	
P03AX01	benzyl benzoate	13.6
R	**RESPIRATORY SYSTEM**	
R01	**Nasal preparations**	
R01A	**Decongestants and other nasal preparations for topical use**	
R01AA	*Sympathomimetics, plain*	
R01AA07	xylometazoline	28
R01AD	*Corticosteroids*	
R01AD05	budesonide	28
R03	**Drugs for obstructive airway diseases**	
R03A	**Adrenergics, inhalants**	
R03AC	*Selective beta-2-adrenoreceptor agonists*	
R03AC02	salbutamol	25.1
R03B	**Other drugs for obstructive airway diseases, inhalants**	
R03BA	*Glucocorticoids*	
R03BA01	beclometasone	25.1
R03BB	*Anticholinergics*	
R03BB01	ipratropium bromide	25.1

ATC code	ATC group/medicine or item	Section
R03C	**Adrenergics for systemic use**	
R03CA	*Alpha- and beta-adrenoreceptor agonists*	
R03CA02	ephedrine	1.2
R03CC	*Selective beta-2-adrenoreceptor agonists*	
R03CC02	salbutamol	25.1
R05	**Cough and cold preparations**	
R05D	**Cough suppressants, excl. combinations with expectorants**	
R05DA	*Opium alkaloids and derivatives*	
R05DA04	codeine	2.2
R06	**Antihistamines for systemic use**	
R06A	**Antihistamines for systemic use**	
R06AB	*Substituted alkylamines*	
R06AB04	chlorphenamine	3
R07	**Other respiratory system products**	
R07A	**Other respiratory system products**	
R07AA	*Lung surfactants*	29
S	**SENSORY ORGANS**	
S01	**Ophthalmologicals**	
S01A	**Antiinfectives**	
S01AA	*Antibiotics*	
S01AA09	tetracycline	21.1
S01AA11	gentamicin	21.1
S01AD	*Antivirals*	
S01AD03	aciclovir	21.1
S01B	**Antiinflammatory agents**	
S01BA	*Corticosteroids, plain*	
S01BA04	prednisolone	21.2
S01E	**Antiglaucoma preparations and miotics**	
S01EA	*Sympathomimetics in glaucoma therapy*	
S01EA01	epinephrine	21.5
S01EB	*Parasympathomimetics*	
S01EB01	pilocarpine	21.4
S01EC	*Carbonic anhydrase inhibitors*	
S01EC01	acetazolamide	21.4

ATC code	ATC group/medicine or item	Section
S01ED	*Beta blocking agents*	
S01ED01	timolol	21.4
S01F	**Mydriatics and cycloplegics**	
S01FA	*Anticholinergics*	
S01FA01	atropine	21.5
S01FA06	tropicamide	14.1
S01H	**Local anesthetics**	
S01HA	*Local anesthetics*	
S01HA03	tetracaine	21.3
S01J	**Diagnostic agents**	
S01JA	*Colouring agents*	
S01JA01	fluorescein	14.1
S02	**Otologicals**	
S02A	**Antiinfectives**	
S02AA	*Antiinfectives*	
S02AA10	acetic acid	28
S02AA15	ciprofloxacin	28
V	**VARIOUS**	
V03	**All other therapeutic products**	
V03A	**All other therapeutic products**	
V03AB	*Antidotes*	
V03AB03	edetates*	4.2
V03AB06	thiosulfate*	4.2; 13.1
V03AB08	sodium nitrite	4.2
V03AB09	dimercaprol	4.2
V03AB14	protamine*	10.2
V03AB15	naloxone	4.2
V03AB17	methylthioninium chloride (methylene blue)	4.2
V03AB23	acetylcysteine	4.2
V03AB31	potassium ferric hexacyanoferrate (II) ·2H2O (Prussian blue)	4.2
V03AC	*Iron chelating agents*	
V03AC01	deferoxamine	4.2; 10.3
V03AF	*Detoxifying agents for antineoplastic treatment*	
V03AF01	mesna	8.2
V03AF03	calcium folinate	8.2

ATC code	ATC group/medicine or item	Section
V03AN	*Medical gases*	
V03AN01	oxygen	1.1.1
V04	**Diagnostic agents**	
V04C	**Other diagnostic agents**	
V04CF	*Tuberculosis diagnostics*	
V04CF01	tuberculin, purified protein derivative (PPD)*	19.1
V07	**All other non-therapeutic products**	
V07A	**All other non-therapeutic products**	
V07AB	*Solvents and diluting agents, incl. irrigating solutions**	26.3
V07AV	*Technical disinfectants**	15.2
V08	**Contrast media**	
V08A	**X-ray contrast media, iodinated**	
V08AA	*Watersoluble, nephrotropic, high osmolar X-ray contrast media*	
V08AA01	diatrizoic acid*	14.2
V08AB	*Watersoluble, nephrotropic, low osmolar X-ray contrast media*	
V08AB02	iohexol	14.2
V08AC	*Watersoluble, hepatotropic X-ray contrast media*	
V08AC02	iotroxic acid*	14.2
V08B	**X-ray contrast media, non-iodinated**	
V08BA	*Barium sulfate containing X-ray contrast media*	
V08BA01	barium sulfate with suspending agents*	14.2

* Medicine or item name differs slightly from the name used.

Annex 4

Alphabetical list of essential medicines (with ATC classification code numbers)

Medicine or item as in EML	ATC code	section
abacavir (ABC)	J05AF06	6.4.2.1
acetazolamide	S01EC01	21.4
acetic acid	S02AA10	28
acetylcysteine	V03AB23	4.2
acetylsalicylic acid	B01AC06	12.5
acetylsalicylic acid	N02BA01	2.1; 7.1
aciclovir	J05AB01	6.4.1
aciclovir	S01AD03	21.1
albendazole	P02CA03	6.1.1; 6.1.2
alcuronium	M03AA01	20
allopurinol	M04AA01	2.3
amidotrizoate*	V08AA01	14.2
amikacin	J01GB06	6.2.4
amiloride	C03DB01	16
amiodarone	C01BD01	12.2
amitriptyline	N06AA09	24.2.1
amlodipine	C08CA01	12.3
amodiaquine	P01BA06	6.5.3.1
amoxicillin	J01CA04	6.2.1
amoxicillin + clavulanic acid*	J01CR02	6.2.1
amphotericin B	J02AA01	6.3; 6.5.2
ampicillin	J01CA01	6.2.1
anti-D immunoglobulin (human)	J06BB01	19.2
antitetanus immunoglobulin (human)	J06BB02	19.2
antivenom immunoglobulin*	J06AA03	19.2
artemether	P01BE02	6.5.3.1
artemether + lumefantrine*	P01BE52	6.5.3.1
artesunate	P01BE03	6.5.3.1
ascorbic acid	A11GA01	27
asparaginase	L01XX02	8.2
atazanavir	J05AE08	6.4.2.3
atenolol	C07AB03	12.1;12.2;12.3
atropine	A03BA01	1.3; 4.2

Medicine or item as in EML	ATC code	section
atropine	S01FA01	21.5
atracurium	M03AC04	20
azathioprine	L04AX01	2.4; 8.1
azithromycin	J01FA10	6.2.2
barium sulfate*	V08BA01	14.2
BCG vaccine*	J07AN01	19.3
beclometasone	R03BA01	25.1
benzathine benzylpenicillin	J01CE08	6.2.1
benznidazole	P01CA02	6.5.5.2
benzoyl peroxide	D10AE01	13.5
benzyl benzoate	P03AX01	13.6
benzylpenicillin	J01CE01	6.2.1
betamethasone	D07AC01	13.3
biperiden	N04AA02	9
bisoprolol	C07AB07	12.1; 12.2; 12.3; 12.4
bleomycin	L01DC01	8.2
budesonide	R01AD05	28
bupivacaine	N01BB01	1.2
caffeine citrate	N06BC01	29
calamine lotion*	D02AB	13.3
calcium folinate	V03AF03	8.2
calcium gluconate	A12AA03	4.2; 27
capreomycin	J04AB30	6.2.4
carbamazepine	N03AF01	5; 24.2.2
carboplatin	L01XA02	8.2
cefalexin	J01DB01	6.2.1
cefazolin	J01DB04	6.2.1
cefixime	J01DD08	6.2.1
cefotaxime	J01DD01	6.2.1
ceftazidime	J01DD02	6.2.1
ceftriaxone	J01DD04	6.2.1
charcoal, activated*	A07BA01	4.1
chlorambucil	L01AA02	8.2
chloramphenicol	J01BA01	6.2.2
chlorhexidine	D08AC02	15.1
chlorine base compound*	D08AX	15.2
chloroquine	P01BA01	2.4; 6.5.3.1; 6.5.3.2
chloroxylenol	D08AE05	15.2

Medicine or item as in EML	ATC code	section
chlorphenamine	R06AB04	3
chlorpromazine	N05AA01	24.1
cholecalciferol*	A12AX	27
cholera vaccine	J07AE	19.3
ciclosporin	L04AA01	8.1
ciprofloxacin	J01MA02	6.2.2
ciprofloxacin	S02AA15	28
clarithromycin	J01FA09	6.2.2
clindamycin	J01FF01	6.2.2
clofazimine	J04BA01	6.2.3
clomifene	G03GB02	18.6
clomipramine	N06AA04	24.4
clotrimazole	G01AF02	6.3
cloxacillin	J01CF02	6.2.1
coal tar*	D05AA	13.5
codeine	R05DA04	2.2
copper-containing device*	G02BA02	18.3.3
cyclophosphamide	L01AA01	8.2
cycloserine	J04AB01	6.2.4
cytarabine	L01BC01	8.2
dacarbazine	L01AX04	8.2
dactinomycin	L01DA01	8.2
dapsone	J04BA02	6.2.3
daunorubicin	L01DB02	8.2
deferoxamine	V03AC01	4.2; 10.3
dexamethasone	H02AB02	3; 8.3; 17.2
dextran 70*	B05AA05	11.1
diaphragms*	G02BB	18.3.4
diazepam	N05BA01	5; 24.3
didanosine (ddI)	J05AF02	6.4.2.1
diethylcarbamazine	P02CB02	6.1.2
digoxin	C01AA05	12.2; 12.4
diloxanide	P01AC01	6.5.1
dimercaprol	V03AB09	4.2
diphtheria antitoxin	J06AA01	19.2
diphtheria vaccine*	J07AF01	19.3
dithranol	D05AC01	13.5
docetaxel	L01CD02	8.2
dopamine	C01CA04	12.4

Medicine or item as in EML	ATC code	section
doxorubicin	L01DB01	8.2
doxycycline	J01AA02	6.2.2; 6.5.3.1; 6.5.3.2
efavirenz (EFV or EFZ)	J05AG03	6.4.2.2
efavirenz + emtricitabine + tenofovir	J05AR06	
eflornithine	P01CX03	6.5.5.1
emtricitabine	J05AF09	6.4.2.1
emtricitabine + tenofovir	J05AR03	
enalapril	C09AA02	12.3; 12.4
ephedrine	R03CA02	1.2
epinephrine (adrenaline)*	S01EA01	21.5
epinephrine (adrenaline)*	C01CA24	3; 12.2; 25.1
ergocalciferol	A11CC01	27
ergometrine	G02AB03	22.1
erythromycin	J01FA01	6.2.2
estradiol cypionate + medroxyprogesterone*	G03AA08	18.3.2
ethambutol	J04AK02	6.2.4
ethambutol + isoniazid*	J04AM03	6.2.4
ethambutol + isoniazid + pyrazinamide + rifampicin*	J04AM06	6.2.4
ethambutol + isoniazid + rifampicin	J04AM	6.2.4
ethanol	D08AX08	15.1
ethinylestradiol + levonorgestrel*	G03AB03	18.3.1
ethinylestradiol + norethisterone*	G03AA05	18.3.1
ethionamide	J04AD03	6.2.4
ethosuximide	N03AD01	5
etoposide	L01CB01	8.2
factor IX complex (coagulation factors II, VII, IX, X) concentrate*	B02BD01	11.2
factor VIII concentrate*	B02BD02	11.2
ferrous salt*	B03A	10.1
ferrous salt + folic acid*	B03AD	10.1
fluconazole	J02AC01	6.3
flucytosine	J02AX01	6.3
fludrocortisone	H02AA02	18.1
fluorescein	S01JA01	14.1
fluorouracil	L01BC02	8.2; 13.5
fluoxetine	N06AB03	24.2.1
fluphenazine	N05AB02	24.1

Medicine or item as in EML	ATC code	section
folic acid	B03BB01	10.1
furosemide	C03CA01	12.4; 16
gentamicin	J01GB03	6.2.2
gentamicin	S01AA11	21.1
glibenclamide	A10BB01	18.5
glucagon	H04AA01	18.5
glucose*	B05BA03	26.2
glucose with sodium chloride*	B05BB02	26.2
glutaral*	V07AV	15.2
glyceryl trinitrate	C01DA02	12.1
griseofulvin	D01BA01	6.3
haemophilus influenzae type b vaccine	J07CA04	19.3
haloperidol	N05AD01	24.1
halothane	N01AB01	1.1.1
heparin sodium*	B01AB01	10.2
hepatitis A vaccine	J07BC02	19.3
hepatitis B vaccine	J07BC01	19.3
human normal immunoglobulin	J06BA	11.2
hydrazaline	C02DB02	12.3
hydrochlorothiazide	C03AA03	12.3; 12.4; 16
hydrocortisone	A07EA02	17.3
hydrocortisone	D07AA02	13.3
hydrocortisone	H02AB09	3; 8.3
hydroxocobalamin	B03BA03	10.1
hydroxycarbamide	L01XX05	8.2; 10.3
ibuprofen	M01AE01	2.1; 29
ifosfamide	L01AA06	8.2
imipenem + cilastatin*	J01DH51	6.2.1
indinavir (IDV)	J05AE02	6.4.2.3
influenza vaccine	J07BB	19.3
insulin injection (soluble)*	A10AB	18.5
intermediate-acting insulin*	A10AC	18.5
intraperitoneal dialysis solution*	B05DA	23
iodine*	A12CX	27
iohexol	V08AB02	14.2
ipratropium bromide	R03BB01	25.1
isoflurane	N01AB06	1.1.1

Medicine or item as in EML	ATC code	section
isoniazid	J04AC01	6.2.4
isoniazid + pyrazinamide + rifampicin*	J04AM05	6.2.4
isoniazid + rifampicin*	J04AM02	6.2.4
isosorbide dinitrate	C01DA08	12.1
ivermectin	P02CF01	6.1.2
Japanese encephalitis vaccine	J07BA02	19.3
kanamycin	J01GB04	6.2.4
ketamine	N01AX03	1.1.2
lamivudine (3TC)	J05AF05	6.4.2.1
lamivudine + nevirapine + stavudine	J05AR07	6.4.2
lamivudine + nevirapine + zidovudine	J05AR05	6.4.2
lamivudine + zidovudine (ZDV or AZT)	J05AR01	6.4.2
levamisole	P02CE01	6.1.1
levodopa + carbidopa*	N04BA02	9
levonorgestrel	G03AC03	18.3.1
levonorgestrel-releasing implant*	G02BA03	18.3.5
levothyroxine*	H03AA01	18.8
lidocaine	C01BB01	12.2
lidocaine	N01BB02	1.2
lidocaine + epinephrine (adrenaline)*	N01BB52	1.2
lithium carbonate*	N05AN01	24.2.2
lopinavir + ritonavir (LPV/r)*	J05AE30	6.4.2.3
lorazepam	N05BA06	5
Lugol's solution*	H03CA	18.8
magnesium sulfate	B05XA05	5
mannitol	B05BC01	16
measles vaccine*	J07BD	19.3
mebendazole	P02CA01	6.1.1
medroxyprogesterone acetate*	G03AC06	18.7
mefloquine	P01BC02	6.5.3.1; 6.5.3.2
meglumine antimoniate	P01CB01	6.5.2
meglumine iotroxate*	V08AC02	14.2
melarsoprol	P01CD01	6.5.5.1
meningococcal meningitis vaccine*	J07AH	19.3
mercaptopurine	L01BB02	8.2
mesna	V03AF01	8.2
metformin	A10BA02	18.5

Medicine or item as in EML	ATC code	section
methadone	N07BC02	24.5
methotrexate	L01BA01	2.4; 8.2
methyldopa*	C02AB01	12.3
methylthioninium chloride (methylene blue)	V03AB17	4.2
metoclopramide	A03FA01	17.2
metronidazole	J01XD01	6.2.2
metronidazole	P01AB01	6.5.1
miconazole	D01AC02	13.1
midazolam	N05CD08	1.3
mifepristone	G03XB01	22.1
miltefosine	L01XX09	6.5.2
misoprostol	G02AD06	22.1
morphine	N02AA01	1.3; 2.2
mumps vaccine	J07BE01	19.3
mupirocin	D06AX09	13.2
naloxone	V03AB15	4.2
neostigmine	N07AA01	20
nevirapine (NVP)	J05AG01	6.4.2.2
niclosamide	P02DA01	6.1.1
nicotinamide	A11HA01	27
nicotine replacement therapy*	N07BA01	24.5
nifedipine	C08CA05	22.2
nifurtimox	P01CC01	6.5.5.1; 6.5.5.2
nitrofurantoin	J01XE01	6.2.2
nitrous oxide	N01AX13	1.1
norethisterone enantate*	G03AC01	18.3.2
nystatin	D01AA01	6.3
ofloxacin	J01MA01	6.2.4
omeprazole	A02BC01	17.1
ondansetron	A04AA01	17.2
oral rehydration salts*	A07CA	17.5.1; 26.1
oxamniquine	P02BA02	6.1.3
oxygen	V03AN01	1.1.1
oxytocin	H01BB02	22.1
paclitaxel	L01CD01	8.2
p-aminosalicylic acid*	J04AA01	6.2.4
pancreatic enzymes	A09AA02	17

Medicine or item as in EML	ATC code	section
paracetamol	N02BE01	2.1; 7.1
paromomycin	A07AA06	6.5.2
penicillamine	M01CC01	2.4; 4.2
pentamidine*	P01CX01	6.5.4; 6.5.5.1
permethrin	P03AC04	13.6
pertussis vaccine	J07AJ	19.3
phenobarbital	N03AA02	5
phenoxymethylpenicillin	J01CE02	6.2.1
phenytoin	N03AB02	5
phytomenadione	B02BA01	10.2
pilocarpine	S01EB01	21.4
pneumoccocal vaccine	J07AL	19.3
podophyllum resin*	D06BB04	13.5
poliomyelitis vaccine	J07BF	19.3
polyvidone iodine	D08AG02	15.1
potassium chloride	B05XA01	26.1; 26.2
potassium ferric hexacyanoferrate (II).$2H_2O$ (Prussian blue)	V03AB31	4.2
potassium iodide*	H03CA	18.8
potassium permanganate	D08AX06	13.2
praziquantel	P02BA01	6.1.1; 6.1.3
prednisolone	H02AB06	3; 8.3
prednisolone	S01BA04	21.2
primaquine	P01BA03	6.5.3.1
procaine benzylpenicillin	J01CE09	6.2.1
procarbazine	L01XB01	8.2
proguanil	P01BB01	6.5.3.2
propofol	N01AX10	1.1.2
propranolol	C07AA05	7.2
propylthiouracil	H03BA02	18.8
prostaglandin E*	C01EA01	29
protamine sulfate*	V03AB14	10.2
pyrantel	P02CC01	6.1.1
pyrazinamide	J04AK01	6.2.4
pyridostigmine	N07AA02	20
pyridoxine	A11HA02	27
pyrimethamine	P01BD01	6.5.4
quinine	P01BC01	6.5.3.1

Medicine or item as in EML	ATC code	section
rabies immunoglobulin	J06BB05	19.2
rabies vaccine	J07BG	19.3
ranitidine	A02BA02	17.1
retinol	A11CA01	27
ribavirin	J05AB04	6.4.3
riboflavin	A11HA04	27
rifabutin	J04AB04	6.2.4
rifampicin	J04AB02	6.2.3; 6.2.4
ritonavir (r)	J05AE03	6.4.2.3
rotavirus vaccine	J07BH01	19.3
rubella vaccine	J07BJ01	19.3
salbutamol	R03AC02	25.1
salbutamol	R03CC02	25.1
salicylic acid	D01AE12	13.5
saquinavir (SQV)	J05AE01	6.4.2.3
selenium sulfide	D01AE13	13.1
senna*	A06AB06	17.4
silver sulfadiazine	D06BA01	13.2
simvastatin	C01AA01	12.6
sodium calcium edetate*	V03AB03	4.2
sodium chloride	B05XA03	26.2
sodium fluoride	A12CD01	27
sodium hydrogen carbonate*	B05XA02	26.2
sodium lactate*	B05BB01	26.2
sodium nitrite	V03AB08	4.2
sodium nitroprusside*	C02DD01	12.3
sodium stibogluconate	P01CB02	6.5.2
sodium thiosulfate*	V03AB06	4.2; 13.1
spectinomycin	J01XX04	6.2.2
spironolactone	C03DA01	16
stavudine (d4T)	J05AF04	6.4.2.1
streptokinase	B01AD01	12.5
streptomycin	J01GA01	6.2.4
succimer	V03AC	4.2
sulfadiazine	J01EC02	6.5.4
sulfadoxine + pyrimethamine*	P01BD51	6.5.3.1
sulfamethoxazole + trimethoprim	J01EE01	6.2.2; 6.5.4
sulfasalazine	A07EC01	2.4; 17.3
suramin sodium	P01CX02	6.5.5.1

Medicine or item as in EML	ATC code	section
surfactant*	R07AA	29
suxamethonium	M03AB01	20
tamoxifen	L02BA01	8.3
tenofovir disoproxil fumarate*	J05AF07	6.4.2.1
terbinafine	D01BA02	13.1
testosterone	G03BA03	18.2
tetanus vaccine	J07AM	19.3
tetracaine	S01HA03	21.3
tetracycline	S01AA09	21.1
thiamine	A11DA01	27
timolol	S01ED01	21.4
tranexamic acid	B02AA02	10.2
triclabendazole	P02BX04	6.1.3
trimethoprim	J01EA01	6.2.2
tropicamide	S01FA06	14.1
tuberculin, purified protein derivative (PPD)*	V04CF01	19.1
typhoid vaccine	J07AP	19.3
urea*	D02AE01	13.5
valproic acid	N03AG01	5; 24.2.2
vancomycin	J01XA01	6.2.2
varicella vaccine	J07BK01	19.3
vecuronium	M03AC03	20
verapamil	C08DA01	12.1; 12.2
vinblastine	L01CA01	8.2
vincristine	L01CA02	8.2
warfarin	B01AA03	10.2
water for injection*	V07AB	26.3
xylometazoline	R01AA07	28
yellow fever vaccine	J07BL	19.3
zidovudine (ZDV or AZT)	J05AF01	6.4.2.1
zinc sulfate	A12CB01	17.5.2

* Medicine or item name differs slightly from the name used.

Annex 5

Report of the Supplementary Meeting of the Expert Committee on the Selection and Use of Essential Medicines

List of participants

Members of the Committee:

Dr Lisa A Bero (Chair), Professor, University of California San Francisco, San Francisco, CA, USA

Dr Gregory L Kearns, Professor of Pediatrics and Pharmacology, University of Missouri Kansas City (UMKC), Kansas City, MO, USA

Mr Andy Gray (Rapporteur), Department of Therapeutics and Medicines Management, Nelson R. Mandela School of Medicine, University of KwaZulu-Natal, Congella, South Africa

Member of the Committee participating via video conference:

Professor Rohini Fernandopulle, Department of Pharmacology, Faculty of Medicine, University of Colombo, Colombo, Sri Lanka

Members of the Committee participating via audio conference:

Professor Noël Cranswick, Clinical Pharmacologist, Royal Children's Hospital/APPRU, Parkville, Victoria, Australia

Dr Alar Irs, Deputy Director, Ravimiamet/State Agency of Medicines, Tartu, Estonia

Professor Anita Zaidi, Associate Professor, Department of Pediatrics and Microbiology, Aga Khan University, Karachi, Pakistan

WHO/HQ:

Dr Hans V Hogerzeil, Director, HSS/EMP

Dr Lembit Rägo, EMP/QSM

Dr Clive Ondari, Coordinator, HSS/EMP/MAR

Dr Suzanne Hill, Secretary, Expert Committee on the Selection and Use of Essential Medicines

Dr Hermann Garden, HSS/EMP/MAR

Dr Catherine d'Arcangues, RHR

Dr Matthews Mathai, MPS

Dr Nikki Shindo, GIP

Dr Charles Penn, GIP

Dr Faith McLellan, HEA

Declaration of interests

All members of the Expert Committee completed the standard WHO form for declaration of interests prior to the meeting. At the start of the meeting, all participants were asked to confirm their interests, and to provide any additional information relevant to the subject matter of the meeting.

The following interests were declared:

Mr Andy Gray reported having accepted travel support from AstraZeneca, Fresenius Kabi, and Aspen Pharmacare to attend continuing education events as a guest speaker, and also receiving research support grants from various donors of antiretroviral medicines used in ACTG and IMPAACT trials and from Gilead Sciences. He also reported being a member of the Scheduling and Naming Expert Committee of the South African Medicines Control Council and being a director of a government funding agency for biotechnology. These were not considered conflicts of interest in relation to the subject of the meeting.

Dr Gregory L Kearns reported being the principal investigator on a NIH grant to Children's Mercy Hospital for projects not related to antivirals and being a Member, Clinical Pharmacology Advisory Committee, Food and Drug Administration, Department of Health and Human Services, USA. These were not considered conflicts of interest in relation to the subject of the meeting.

Dr Anita Zaidi reported receiving research funding in the past three years from Wyeth in the area of pneumococcal surveillance for her research unit, now completed. This was not considered a conflict of interest in relation to the subject of the meeting.

Dr Lisa A Bero, Professor Noël Cranswick, Professor Rohini Fernandopulle, and Dr Alar Irs reported no conflicts of interest.

Introduction

A Supplementary Meeting of the WHO Expert Committee on the Selection and Use of Essential Medicines took place in Geneva on 15 January 2010.

The meeting was opened on behalf of the Director-General by Dr Hans V Hogerzeil, Director of the Department of Essential Medicines and Pharmaceutical Policies (EMP). He stated that the evidence in relation to essential medicines is changing rapidly and that WHO needs to consider this when planning its activities. He further noted that this session was the first ever supplementary session of the Expert Committee, following approval in principle by the Director-General of the proposals for such meetings from the March 2009 meeting. He noted that apart from the shortened timeline, the main change to the normal committee meeting processes was the use of telephone/video conference links to hold the meeting. All other procedures for the Expert Committee had been followed, including posting documents on the WHO web site, together with the rounds of review and comments prior to the meeting.

Dr Hogerzeil briefly explained some aspects of the Committee procedures. He stated that the Committee is not a representative one; all members participate in their own personal capacity and are not allowed to take instructions from any government or any other authority. He also noted the increasing attention being paid to potential conflicts of interest in relation, in particular, to influenza policies and expressed confidence in the procedures followed in regard to this meeting. The Committee followed its usual procedures in relation to reporting and evaluation of conflicts of interest of members, as summarized in this report.

Section 6.4.3: Other antiviral medicines

Amantadine and rimantadine, oseltamivir, zanamivir (Inclusion)

At its March meeting in 2009, the Expert Committee considered four applications for antivirals to be included in the WHO Model List of Essential Medicines: amantadine, rimantadine, oseltamivir, and zanamivir.

The Committee's decisions at that meeting were:

> The Committee noted that the costs of amantadine and rimantadine vary but are generally cheaper than the neuraminidase inhibitors. Overall the evidence to support the effectiveness of any of the four antivirals for treatment of avian influenza remains very low quality. The effect of these medicines on seasonal influenza is better established, but may be of less importance. When used for treatment of individual cases of

> H5N1, the cost is low but in the context of seasonal influenza, they have not been accepted as cost effective. On balance, the potential advantage of the inclusion of any of them on the List would be to perhaps increase availability and decrease price. This would be critical in the context of responding to a pandemic, but the pandemic preparedness plans already include stockpiling of antivirals (often donated.) It is not clear that addition of the medicines to the List would enhance this access programme.
>
> After consideration of these factors, the Committee recommended not including any of the antivirals on the List at the present time. However the Committee endorsed the proposal for an emergency meeting mechanism to consider one or more, including for paediatric use, should a pandemic occur.

The situation since the March 2009 meeting has changed, in that a pandemic has indeed occurred. The pandemic influenza virus, pH1N1, is sensitive to neuraminidase inhibitors, but not to the M2 inhibitors. There has been considerable debate about the role of oseltamivir and zanamivir in treatment and prophylaxis of infection due to the pandemic virus, which has for the present almost completely replaced seasonal influenza virus as the main circulating strain.

WHO issued treatment guidelines in August 2009 that recommended use of oseltamivir and zanamivir for treatment in certain patient groups, particularly for those patients presenting with complications or severe disease. This recommendation was based on assessment of the randomized trial data represented to the Expert Committee in March 2009, plus an evaluation of observational studies that suggest that antivirals may reduce the rate of clinically relevant complications of influenza. In those guidelines, oseltamivir was considered as the first option for treatment.

An update of these guidelines and the draft recommendations from the guideline panel, which met on 13–14 January 2010, were provided to the Expert Committee. The updated evidence summaries prepared for the guideline meeting, including the GRADE evidence profiles summarizing available evidence, were also provided to the Expert Committee.

Since March 2009, the registration information for oseltamivir and zanamivir for use in children has been amended by both the US Food and Drug Administration and the European Medicines Agency. Generic versions of oseltamivir have been registered in a number of countries and a number of oseltamivir products have been prequalified for United Nations procurement by WHO. There have been no changes in the regulatory status to amantadine and rimantadine as far as the Committee has been able to determine.

Evidence summary

A full update of the evidence available in relation to the four antivirals, including observational studies (*393–397*) relating to use of the antivirals in the context of the pandemic has been prepared for the guideline panel and circulated to the Committee. The Committee noted the following:

- There are no new data from randomized trials for any of the four antivirals under consideration.
- The majority of randomized trials are in the healthy adult population; there is one systematic review of trials in children (*398*).
- The majority of the randomized trials do not report clinically relevant outcomes such as development of pneumonia, hospitalization, or mortality. The only published analysis with these data is a report of a pooled analysis from a set of data from Roche [published as Kaiser et al. (*399*)]. This study was excluded from the update of the Cochrane Review [published as Jefferson et al. (*400*)] as the data from all of the individual trials were not made available to the authors of the Cochrane Review. The exclusion of this study and the possibility of publication bias in the trials conducted by Roche has been the subject of discussion in the *British Medical Journal* articles (*401–403*) published with the Cochrane Review.
- The observational data are summarized in the updated evidence summary for the guideline panel (*404–406*) and also in various studies (*407–416*), and, in the population studied – including higher-risk groups – suggest a significant benefit of treatment with oseltamivir in terms of reduction of hospitalization and occurrence of pneumonia. Three observational studies (*404*, *415*, *417*) suggest benefit in terms of reduction in mortality. There are fewer data for zanamivir and no current observational studies of amantadine or rimantadine that are relevant.
- Adverse effects of all four antivirals are well characterized. The only additional data from March 2009 was the observation that the neuropsychiatric effects that have been reported in relation to oseltamivir have not been reported so far in studies outside of Japan, notwithstanding extensive use in a number of countries over the past six months.
- The data from children have been summarized in the evidence update. In addition, an unpublished analysis by Abdel-Rahman and Kearns of information relating to dosing of oseltamivir in children aged less than two years has been provided for the guideline panel.

Considerations of the Expert Committee

The Committee noted that there was no change to the cost and availability information for amantadine and rimantadine from March 2009. With respect to oseltamivir, it was noted that the cost had generally come down and was variable as multiple manufacturers have registered and also prequalified products through the WHO–UN programme, and donation programmes are in place. For zanamivir, no change in cost or the low availability of the inhaled preparation was noted, although this medicine is also included in the WHO–UN Prequalification Programme expression of interest and at least one product has been prequalified. The Committee was informed that an intravenous preparation of zanamivir was available in a limited number of countries as an experimental product, but it was not yet licensed anywhere.

The comments received from Expert Panel members and others on the proposals posted on the web site were noted by the Committee. Generally, the comments highlighted the absence of RCT evidence directly relating to the evidence for effectiveness and safety of all antivirals in the pandemic, as well as raising questions about whether any antiviral would meet the definition of an essential medicine.

The Committee considered that:

The evidence from RCTs for all antivirals has not changed substantially since March 2009. However, there has been more experience of the use of oseltamivir since the declaration of the pandemic, and the observational data resulting from this use provide some estimates of effectiveness. Since March 2009, there is also more evidence of the relative safety of oseltamivir in a range of patient and age groups, with no evidence of harm. The updated WHO recommendations concerning use of oseltamivir for treatment of seriously ill patients or those in higher-risk groups are based on these data. Oseltamivir resistance has been described, very rarely, for the current pandemic H1N1 strain. In these cases, the virus has remained susceptible to zanamivir. However, there remain concerns that increasing use of antivirals will lead to increased resistance.

Based on the available evidence of the potential benefit of oseltamivir in specific patient groups and the expected prevalence of pandemic H1N1 in the coming seasons, the Expert Committee agreed to add this medicine to the Core List. The Committee specified that the List should include the following notes: oseltamivir should be used only in compliance with the WHO treatment guidelines, i.e. (1) for treatment of patients with severe or progressive clinical illness with confirmed or suspected influenza pandemic (H1N1); and (2) for the treatment of patients with confirmed or suspected but uncomplicated illness due to pandemic influenza virus infection who were in higher-risk groups, most notably pregnant women and children aged less than 2 years.

Oseltamivir will be listed in the following dosage forms:

- Capsule: 30 mg; 45 mg; 75 mg.
- Oral powder: 12 mg/ml.

The Committee noted the ongoing need for age-appropriate dosage forms for children, including neonates.

The WHO treatment guidelines will be reviewed in the early Northern winter of 2010, and the Committee therefore recommended that its decision to include oseltamivir should be reviewed at the March 2011 scheduled meeting of the Expert Committee. This scheduled review will also be noted in the EML.

Evidence for benefits of zanamivir in this pandemic is very limited and in the current situation, amantadine and rimantadine are ineffective. The Committee therefore decided not to include zanamivir, as currently, it may only be required in a limited number of circumstances, such as in patients who are found to have infection due to pandemic H1N1 that is resistant to oseltamivir. The evidence for its effectiveness was considerably less than the evidence for oseltamivir. The inhaled dosage form is also more difficult to use in patients presenting with severe or progressive illness and cannot be used in children aged less than 5 years.

The Committee confirmed the decision of March 2009 in relation to amantadine and rimantadine, and recommended that they should not be included on the WHO Model List of Essential Medicines.

In closing the meeting, the Chair noted that the report of the meeting would be circulated electronically to all members of the Committee for ratification, and it would then be submitted for the usual WHO approval processes by the Secretariat.

References

1. Orme et al. Clinical pharmacology in research, teaching and health care. Considerations by IUPHAR, the International Union of Basic and Clinical Pharmacology. *Basic and Clinical Pharmacology and Toxicology*, 2010, 107(1):531–559.
2. Pierce CA, Voss B. Efficacy and safety of ibuprofen and acetaminophen in children and adults: a meta-analysis and qualitative review. *The Annals of Pharmacotherapy*, 2010, 44(3):489–506.
3. Eyers S et al. The effect on mortality of antipyretics in the treatment of influenza infection: systematic review and meta-analysis. *Journal of the Royal Society of Medicine*, 2010, 103:403–411.
4. Strengell T et al. Antipyretic agents for preventing recurrences of febrile seizures. *Archives of Pediatrics and Adolescent Medicine*, 2009, 163(9):799–804.
5. Southey ER et al. Systematic review and meta-analysis of the clinical safety and tolerability of ibuprofen compared with paracetamol in paediatric pain and fever. *Current Medical Research and Opinion*, 2009, 25(9):2207–2222.
6. Kanabar DS et al. A review of ibuprofen and acetaminophen use in febrile children and the occurrence of asthma-related symptoms. *Clinical Therapeutics*, 2007, 29(12):2716–2723.
7. Williams DG et al. Codeine phosphate in paediatric medicine. *British Journal of Anaesthesia*, 2001, 86(3):413–421.
8. Clark E et al. A randomized controlled trial of acetaminophen, ibuprofen and codeine for acute pain relief in children with musculoskeletal trauma. *Paediatrics*, 2007, 119:460–467.
9. Ruiz-Irastorza G et al. Clinical efficacy and side effects of antimalarials in systemic lupus erythematosus: a systematic review. *Annals of the Rheumatic Diseases*, 2010, 69(1):20–28.
10. Stringer E et al. Treatment approaches to juvenile dermatomyositis (JDM) across North America: The Childhood Arthritis and Rheumatology Research Alliance (CARRA) JDM Treatment Survey. *The Journal of Rheumatology*, 2010, 37(9):1953–1961.
11. Fujinaga S et al. Maintenance therapy with mycophenolate mofetil for children with severe lupus nephritis after low-dose intravenous cyclophosphamide regimen. *Pediatric Nephrology*, 2008, 23(10):1877–1882.
12. Takken T, Van Der Net J, Helders PJ. Methotrexate for treating juvenile idiopathic arthritis. *Cochrane Database of Systematic Reviews*, 2001, (4):CD003129.
13. Giannini EH et al. Comparative efficacy and safety of advanced drug therapy in children with juvenile rheumatoid arthritis. *Seminars in Arthritis & Rheumatism*, 1993, 23(1):34–46.
14. Ruperto N et al. A randomized trial of parenteral methotrexate comparing an intermediate dose with a higher dose in children with juvenile idiopathic arthritis who failed to respond to standard doses of methotrexate. *Arthritis & Rheumatism*, 2004, 50(7):2191–2201.
15. Huber AM et al. Protocols for the initial treatment of moderately severe juvenile dermatomyositis: results of a Children's Arthritis and Rheumatology Research Alliance Consensus Conference. *Arthritis Care and Research (Hoboken)*, 2010, 62(2):219–225.
16. Holzinger D, Frosch M, Föll D. Methotrexate in the therapy of juvenile idiopathic arthritis. *Zeitschrift für Rheumatologie*, 2010, 69(6):496–504.
17. Singsen BH, Goldbach-Mansky R. Methotrexate in the treatment of juvenile rheumatoid arthritis and other pediatric rheumatoid and nonrheumatic disorders. *Rheumatic Disease Clinics of North America*, 1997, 23(4):811–840.
18. Silverman E et al. Long-term open-label preliminary study of the safety and efficacy of leflunomide in patients with polyarticular-course juvenile rheumatoid arthritis. *Arthritis & Rheumatism*, 2005, 52(2):554–562.

19. van Rossum MA et al. Sulfasalazine in the treatment of juvenile chronic arthritis: a randomized, double-blind, placebo-controlled, multicenter study. Dutch Juvenile Chronic Arthritis Study Group. *Arthritis & Rheumatism*, 1998, 41(5):808–816.
20. Burgos-Vargas R et al. A 26-week randomised, double blind, placebo controlled exploratory study of sulfasalazine in juvenile onset spondyloarthropathies. *Annals of the Rheumatic Diseases*, 2002, 61(10):941–942.
21. Ansell BM et al. A multicentre pilot study of sulphasalazine in juvenile chronic arthritis. *Clinical and Experimental Rheumatology*, 1991, 9(2):201–203.
22. Gerloni V et al. Efficacy and safety profile of cyclosporin A in the treatment of juvenile chronic (idiopathic) arthritis. Results of a 10-year prospective study. *Rheumatology (Oxford)*, 2001, 40(8):907–913.
23. Reiff A et al. Preliminary evidence for cyclosporin A as an alternative in the treatment of recalcitrant juvenile rheumatoid arthritis and juvenile dermatomyositis. *The Journal of Rheumatology*, 1997, 24(12):2436–2443.
24. Kvien TK, Hoyeraal HM, Sandstad B. Azathioprine versus placebo in patients with juvenile rheumatoid arthritis: a single center double blind comparative study. *The Journal of Rheumatology*, 1986, 13(1):118–123.
25. Savolainen HA et al. Azathioprine in patients with juvenile chronic arthritis: a longterm followup study. *The Journal of Rheumatology*, 1997, 24(12):2444–2450.
26. Hagelberg S et al. Longterm followup of childhood lupus nephritis. *The Journal of Rheumatology*, 2002, 29(12):2635–2642.
27. Brewer EJ et al. Penicillamine and hydroxychloroquine in the treatment of severe juvenile rheumatoid arthritis. Results of the U.S.A.-U.S.S.R. double-blind placebo-controlled trial. *The New England Journal of Medicine*, 1986, 314(20):1269–1276.
28. Kvien TK, Hoyeraal HM, Sandstad S. Slow acting antirheumatic drugs in patients with juvenile rheumatoid arthritis — evaluated in a randomized, parallel 50-week clinical trial. *The Journal of Rheumatology*, 1985, 12(3):533–539.
29. Suarez-Almazor ME et al. Antimalarials for treating rheumatoid arthritis. *Cochrane Database of Systematic Reviews*, 2000, (4):CD000959.
30. Brittenham GM. Iron chelating therapy for transfusional iron overload. *The New England Journal of Medicine*, 2011, 364:146–156.
31. Griffith EA et al. Effect of deferasirox on iron absorption in a randomized, placebo-controlled, crossover study in a human model of acute supratherapeutic iron ingestion. *Annals of Emergency Medicine*, 2011, 58(1):69–73.
32. Olivieri NF et al. Survival in medically treated patients with homozygous B-thalassemia. *The New England Journal of Medicine*, 1994, 331:574–578.
33. Zurlo MG et al. Survival and causes of death in thalassaemia major. *The Lancet*, 1989, 2:27–30.
34. Borgna-Pignatti C et al. Survival and complications in patients with thalassemia major treated with transfusion and deferoxamine. *Haematologica*, 2004, 89:1187–1193.
35. Wolfe L et al. Prevention of cardiac disease by subcutaneous deferoxamine in patients with thalassemia major. *The New England Journal of Medicine*, 1985, 312:1600–1603.
36. Brittenham GM et al. Efficacy of deferoxamine in preventing complications of iron overload in patients with thalassemia major. *The New England Journal of Medicine*, 1994, 331:567–573.
37. Roberts D et al. Oral deferiprone for iron chelation in people with thalassemia. *Cochrane Database of Systematic Reviews*, 2007, (3):CD004839.

38. Roberts D et al. Desferrioxamine mesylate for managing transfusional iron overload in people with transfusion-dependent thalassaemia. *Cochrane Database of Systematic Reviews*, 2005, (4):CD004450.

39. Kontoghiorghes GJ. The 18th ICOC proceedings in Athens, Greece: new breakthrough in thalassemia leading to the complete treatment of iron overload and to hundreds of patients achieving and maintaining normal body iron stores. Ethical questions on chelation therapy. *Hemoglobin*, 2010, 34(3):199–203.

40. Tanner MA et al. A randomized, placebo-controlled, double-blind trial of the effect of combined therapy with deferoxamine and deferiprone on myocardial iron in thalassemia major using cardiovascular magnetic resonance. *Circulation*, 2007, 115:1876–1884.

41. Delea TE et al. Cost effectiveness of once-daily oral chelation therapy with deferasirox versus infusional deferoxamine in transfusion-dependent thalassaemia patients: US healthcare system perspective. *Pharmacoeconomics*, 2007, 25:329–342.

42. Chisholm JJ, Thomas DJ. Use of 2,3-dimercaptopropane-1-sulfonate in treatment of lead poisoning in children. *Journal of Pharmacology and Experimental Therapeutics*, 1985, 235:665–669.

43. Bartsocas CS et al: Oral d-penicillamine and intramuscular BAL + EDTA in the treatment of lead accumulation. *Acta paediatrica Scandinavica*, 1971, 60:553–558.

44. Shannon MW, Townsend MK. Adverse effects of reduced d-penicillamine in children with mild to moderate lead poisoning. *The Annals of Pharmacotherapy*, 2000, 34:15–18.

45. Moncrieff AA et al. Lead poisoning in children. *Archives of Disease in Childhood*, 1964, 39:1–13.

46. Glotzer DE, Freedberg KA, Bauchner H. Management of childhood lead poisoning: clinical impact and cost-effectiveness. *Medical Decision Making*, 1995, 15:13–24.

47. TOXBASE. *Lead chelation therapy in children*. United Kingdom National Poisons Information Service, 2009.

48. American Academy of Pediatrics, Committee on Drugs. Treatment guidelines for lead exposure in children. *Pediatrics*, 1995, 96:155–160.

49. *L'intoxication par le plomb de l'enfant et de la femme enceinte*. Guide publié en 2006 par le Ministère de la Santé et des Solidarités, Paris (http://www.sante.gouv.fr/IMG/pdf/guide_depistage_saturnisme-2.pdf, accessed 29 September 2011).

50. Graziano JH et al. Controlled study of meso-2,3-dimercaptosuccinic acid for the management of childhood lead intoxication. *Journal of Pediatrics*, 1992, 120:133–139.

51. Farrar HC et al. A comparison of two dosing regimens of succimer in children with chronic lead poisoning. *The Journal of Clinical Pharmacology*, 1999, 39:180–183.

52. O'Connor ME, Rich D. Children with moderately elevated lead levels: is chelation with DMSA helpful? *Clinical Pediatrics*, 1999, 38:325–331.

53. Rogan WJ et al. Treatment of Lead-Exposed Children Trial Group. The effect of chelation therapy with succimer on neuropsychological development in children exposed to lead. *The New England Journal of Medicine*, 2001, 344(19):1421–1426.

54. Besunder JB et al. Short-term efficacy of oral dimercaptosuccinic acid in children with low to moderate lead intoxication. *Pediatrics*, 1995, 96:683–687.

55. Liebelt EL et al. Efficacy of oral meso-2,3 dimercaptosuccinic acid therapy for low-level childhood plumbism. *Journal of Pediatrics*, 1994, 124:313–317.

56. Graziano JH et al. Dose-response study of oral 2,3-dimercaptosuccinic acid in children with elevated blood lead concentrations. *Journal of Pediatrics*, 1988, 113:751–757.

57. Counter SA et al. Lead concentrations in maternal blood and breast milk and pediatric blood of Andean villagers: 2006 follow-up investigation. *Journal of Occupational and Environmental Medicine*, 2007, 49:302–309.
58. Zavaleta CAS. Support for Phase II of the Peru lead project to determine blood and ambient lead levels in metropolitan Lima and to manage the lead exposure problem in critical areas. Activity Report 110, 2001 (http://www.ehproject.org/PDF/Activity_Reports/AR110-PELeadPrj2Final.pdf, accessed 29 September 2011).
59. Senegal: Outbreak of lead intoxication in Thiaroye sur Mer, Senegal. Geneva, World Health Organization, Update 2-23 February 2009 (http://www.who.int/environmental_health_emergencies/events/Senegal2008_update2/en/index.html, accessed 29 September 2011).
60. *Control of the leishmaniases. Report of a meeting of the WHO Expert Committee on the Control of Leishmaniases*. Geneva, World Health Organization, 2010 (*WHO Technical Report Series, No. 949*).
61. *Working to overcome the global impact of neglected tropical diseases – First WHO report on neglected tropical diseases*. Geneva, World Health Organization, 2010.
62. Stoltzfus RJ et al. Effects of iron supplementation and antihelminthic treatment on motor and language development of preschool children in Zanzibar: double blind, placebo controlled study. *British Medical Journal*, 2001, 323:1–8.
63. Flohr C et al. Low efficacy of mebendazole against hookworm in Vietnam: two randomized controlled trials. *The American Journal of Tropical Medicine and Hygiene*, 2007, 76(4):732–736.
64. Albonico M et al. Efficacy of mebendazole and levamisole alone or in combination against intestinal nematode infections after repeated targeted mebendazole treatment in Zanzibar. *Bulletin of the World Health Organization*, 2003, 81(5):343–352.
65. Montresor A, Awashiti S, Crompton DWT. Use of benzimidazoles in children younger than 24 months for the treatment of soil-transmitted helminthiasis. *Acta Tropica*, 2003, 86:223–232.
66. Albonico M et al. A controlled evaluation of two school-based antihelminthic chemotherapy regimens on intensity of intestinal helminth infections. *International Journal of Epidemiology*, 1999, 28(3):591–596.
67. Sacko M et al. Comparison of the efficacy of mebendazole, albendazole and pyrantel in treatment of human hookworm infections in the Southern region of Mali, West Africa. *Transactions of the Royal Society of Tropical Medicine & Hygiene*, 1999, 93:195–203.
68. Albonico M et al. Evaluation of the efficacy of pyrantel-oxantel for the treatment of soil-transmitted nematode infections. *Transactions of the Royal Society of Tropical Medicine & Hygiene*, 2002, 96:685–690.
69. Cañete R et al. Randomized clinical study of five days therapy with mebendazole compared to quinacrine in the treatment of symptomatic giardiasis in children. *World Journal of Gastroenterology*, 2006, 12(39):6366–6370.
70. Northrop-Clewes CA et al. Antihelminthic treatment of rural Bangladeshi children: effect on host physiology, growth and biochemical status. *American Journal of Clinical Nutrition*, 2001, 73:53–60.
71. Morrone FB et al. Study of enteroparasites infection frequency and chemotherapeutic agents used in pediatric patients in a community living in Porto Alegre, RS, Brazil. *Revista do Instituto de Medicina Tropical de São Paulo*, 2004, 46(2):77–80.
72. Thein-Hlaing, Than Saw, Myat-Lay-Kyin. Control of ascariasis through age targeted chemotherapy: impact of 6-monthly chemotherapeutic regimens. *Bulletin of the World Health Organization*, 1990, 68:747–753.

73. Lionel ND et al. Levamisole in the treatment of ascariasis in children. *British Medical Journal*, 1969, 4:340–341.

74. Forrester JE et al. Randomised trial of albendazole and pyrantel in symptomless trichuriasis in children. *The Lancet*, 1998, 352:1103–1108.

75. Kshirsagar NA et al. Safety, tolerability, efficacy and plasma concentrations of diethylcarbamazine and albendazole co-administration in a field study in an area endemic for lymphatic filariasis in India. *Transactions of the Royal Society of Tropical Medicine & Hygiene*, 2004, 98:205–217.

76. Rizzo J et al. Children and adolescents infected with *Wuchereria bancrofti* in Great Recife, Brazil: a randomized, year long clinical trial of single treatments with diethylcarbamazine or diethylcarbamazine–albendazole. *Annals of Tropical Medicine and Parasitology*, 2007, 101(5):423–433.

77. Ramaiah KD et al. Impact of 10 years of diethlycarbamazine and ivermectin mass administration on infection and transmission of lymphatic filariasis. *Transactions of the Royal Society of Tropical Medicine & Hygiene*, 2007, 101:555–563.

78. Weil GJ et al. The impact of repeated rounds of mass drug administration with diethylcarbamazine plus albendazole on bancroftian filariasis in Papua New Guinea. *PloS Neglected Tropical Diseases*, 2008, 2(12):e344.

79. Babu BV et al. Adverse reactions following mass drug administration during the Programme to Eliminate Lymphatic Filariasis in Orissa State, India. *Transactions of the Royal Society of Tropical Medicine & Hygiene*, 2006, 100:464–469.

80. Ramzy RMR et al. Effect of yearly mass drug administration with diethlcarbamazine and albendazole on bancroftian filariasis in Egypt: a comprehensive assessment. *The Lancet*, 2006, 367:992–999.

81. Beach MJ et al. Assessment of combined ivermectin and albendazole for treatment of intestinal helminth and *Wuchereria bancrofti* infections in Haitian schoolchildren. *American Journal of Tropical Medicine and Hygiene*, 1999, 60(3):479–486.

82. Simonsen PE et al. The effect of single dose ivermectin alone or in combination with albendazole on *Wuchereria bancrofti* infection in primary school children in Tanzania. *Transactions of the Royal Society of Tropical Medicine & Hygiene*, 2004, 98:462–472.

83. Asio SM, Simonsen PE, Onapa AW. A randomised, double-blind field trial of ivermectin alone and in combination with albendazole for the treatment of *Mansonella perstans* infections in Uganda. *Transactions of the Royal Society of Tropical Medicine & Hygiene*, 2009, 103:274–279.

84. Vyungimana F, Newell E. Treatment of onchocerciasis with ivermectin (province of Bururi, Burundi): parasitologic and clinical evaluation of different periodicities of treatment. *American Journal of Tropical Medicine and Hygiene*, 1998, 59(5):828–831.

85. Ndyomugyenyi R et al. The impact of ivermectin treatment alone and when in parallel with *Simulium neavei* elimination on onchocerciasis in Uganda. *Tropical Medicine & International Health*, 2004, 9:882–886.

86. Mohammed KA et al. Triple co-administration of ivermectin, albendazole and praziquantel in Zanzibar: a safety study. *PloS Neglected Tropical Diseases*, 2008, 2(1):e171.

87. Sacko M et al. The effect of single dose versus two doses of praziquantel on *Schistosoma haematobium* infection and pathology among school-aged children in Mali. *Parasitology*, 2009, 136:1851–1857.

88. Ferrari MLA et al. Efficacy of oxamniquine and praziquantel in the treatment of *Schistosoma mansoni* infection: a controlled trial. *Bulletin of the World Health Organization*, 2003, 81:190–196.

89. Sissoko MS et al. Efficacy of artesunate + sulfamethoxypyrazine/pyrimethamine versus praziquantel in the treatment of *Schistosoma haematobium* in children. *PLoS ONE*, 2009, 4(10):e6732.

90. Inyang-Etoh PC et al. Efficacy of a combination of praziquantel and artesunate in the treatment of urinary schistosomiasis in Nigeria. *Transactions of the Royal Society of Tropical Medicine & Hygiene*, 2009, 103:38–44.

91. Hou XY et al. A randomized, double-blind, placebo-controlled trial of safety and efficacy of combined praziquantel and artemether treatment for acute schistosomiasis japonica in China. *Bulletin of the World Health Organization*, 2008, 86:788–795.

92. Nokes C et al. Evidence for an improvement in cognitive function following treatment of *Schistosoma japonicum* infection in Chinese primary school children. *American Journal of Tropical Medicine and Hygiene*, 1999, 60(4):556–565.

93. Pugh RNH, Teesdale CH. Single dose oral treatment in urinary schistosomiasis: a double blind trial. *British Medical Journal*, 1983, 286:429–432.

94. Keiser J et al. Efficacy and safety of mefloquine, artesunate, mefloquine-artesunate, and praziquantel against *Schistosoma haematobium*: Randomized, exploratory open-label trial. *Clinical Infectious Diseases*, 2010, 50(9):1205–1213.

95. Touré S et al. Two-year impact of single praziquantel treatment on infection in the national control programme on schistosomiasis in Burkina Faso. *Bulletin of the World Health Organization*, 2008, 86:780–787.

96. Midzi N et al. Efficacy and side effects of praziquantel treatment against *Schistosoma haematobium* infection among primary school children in Zimbabwe. *Transactions of the Royal Society of Tropical Medicine & Hygiene*, 2008, 102:759–766.

97. Tuchuenté LAT et al. Efficacy of praziquantel against *Schistosoma haematobium* infection in children. *American Journal of Tropical Medicine and Hygiene*, 2004, 7(6):776–782.

98. Davis A, Biles JE, Ulrich AM. Initial experiences with praziquantel in the treatment of human infections due to *Schistosoma haematobium*. *Bulletin of the World Health Organization*, 1979, 57(5):773–779.

99. *Treatment of young children for schistosomiasis in Sudan* (Amin PI et al., unpublished data, 2010).

100. *Treatment of children under 5 years old: an investigation of the accessibility, safety, efficacy and immunology of praziquantel treatment* (Gwisai et al., unpublished data, 2010).

101. *Treatment of intestinal schistosomiasis using praziquantel syrup versus crushed praziquantel tablet in Ugandan preschool children* (Kabatereine et al., unpublished data, 2010).

102. *Assessing tolerance to and efficacy of EPIQUANTEL® syrup (praziquantel) on* S. haematobium *and* S. mansoni *infected pre-school children in Niger* (Garba et al., unpublished data, 2010).

103. *Treatment of primary school children from schistosomiasis mansoni with praziquantel suspension* (Barakat et al., unpublished data, 2010).

104. Ayele T. Preliminary clinical trial of oral oxamniquine in the treatment of *Schistosoma mansoni* in children in Ethiopia. *East African Medical Journal*, 1986, 63(4):291–294.

105. Abdel Rahim IM, Haridi AAM, Abdel-Hameed AA. Field study of different oxamniquine dose for *Schistosoma mansoni* in Gezira, Sudan. *Journal of Tropical Medicine & Hygiene*, 1988, 91:131–137.

106. Kilpatrick ME et al. Oxamniquine versus niridazole for treatment of uncomplicated *Schistosoma mansoni* infection. *The American Journal of Tropical Medicine and Hygiene*, 1982, 31(6):1164–1167.

107. Lambertucci JR et al. A double blind trial with oxamniquine in chronic schistosomiasis mansoni. *Transactions of the Royal Society of Tropical Medicine & Hygiene*, 1982, 76(6):751–755.

108. Axton JHM, Garnett PA. A trial of oral oxamniquine in the treatment of schistosoma infection in children. *South African Medical Journal*, 1976, 50:1051–1053.

109. Katz N, Zicker F, Pereira JP. Field trials with oxamniquine in a schistosomiasis mansoni-endemic area. *The American Journal of Tropical Medicine and Hygiene*, 1977, 26(1):234–237.

110. Katz N et al. Efficacy of alternating therapy with oxamniquine and praziquantel to treat *Schistosoma mansoni* in children following failure of first treatment. *The American Journal of Tropical Medicine and Hygiene*, 1991, 44(5):509–512.

111. Gryseels B, Nkulikyinka L, Coosemans MH. Field trials of praziquantel and oxamniquine for treatment of schistosomiasis mansoni in Burundi. *Transactions of the Royal Society of Tropical Medicine & Hygiene*, 1987, 81:641–44.

112. Gryseels M, Nkulikyinka L. Two-year follow-up of *Schistosoma mansoni* infection and morbidity after treatment with different regimens of oxamniquine and praziquantel. *Transactions of the Royal Society of Tropical Medicine & Hygiene*, 1989, 83:219–228.

113. Hammouda NA et al. Therapeutic effect of tricalbendazole in patients with fascioliasis in Egypt a preliminary study. *Journal of the Egyptian Society of Parasitology*, 1995, 25(1):137–143.

114. El-Morshedy H et al. Triclabendazole in the treatment of human fascioliasis: a community-based study. *La Revue de Santé de la Méditerranée orientale*, 1999, 5(5):888–894.

115. El-Karaksy H et al. Human fascioliasis in Egyptian children: successful treatment with triclabendazole. *Journal of Tropical Pediatrics*, 1999, 45(3):135–139.

116. Ortiz JJ et al. Randomized clinical study of niazoxanide compared to metronidazole in the treatment of symptomatic giardiasis in children from Northern Peru. *Alimentary Pharmacology and Therapeutics*, 2001, 15(9):1409–1415.

117. Dinleyici EC et al. Clinical efficacy of *Saccharomyces boulardii* and metronidazole compared to metronidazole alone in children with acute bloody diarrhea caused by amebiasis: a prospective, randomized, open label study. *The American Journal of Tropical Medicine and Hygiene*, 2009, 80(6):953–955.

118. Talri SA et al. Comparison of metronidazole and furazolidone against *Giardia lamblia* in children. *Journal of Medical Sciences*, 2006, 6(3):378–381.

119. Suntornpoch V, Chavalittamrong B. Treatment of giardiasis in children with tinidazole, ornidazole and metronidazole. *The Southeast Asian Journal of Tropical Medicine and Public Health*, 1981, 12(2):231–235.

120. Sadjjadi SM, Alborzi AW, Mostovfi H. Comparative clinical trial of mebendazole and metronidazole in Giardiasis of children. *Journal of Tropical Pediatrics*, 2001, 47(3):176–178.

121. Rubidge CJ, Scragg JN, Powell SJ. Treatment of children with acute amoebic dysentery: comparative trial of metronidazole against a combination of dehydroemetine, tetracycline and diloxanide furoate. *Archives of Disease in Childhood*, 1970, 45:196–197.

122. McAuley JB et al. Diloxanide furoate for treating asymptomatic *Entamoeba histolytica* cyst passers: 14 years' experience in the United States. *Clinical Infectious Diseases*, 1992, 15(3):464–468.

123. Balasegaram M et al. Treatment outcomes and risk factors for relapse in patients with early-stage human African typanonsomiasis (HAT) in the Republic of the Congo. *Bulletin of the World Health Organization*, 2006, 84:777–782.

124. Blum JA et al. Cardiac alterations in human African trypanosomiasis (*T.b.gambiense*) with respect to the disease stage and antiparasitic treatment. *PloS Neglected Tropical Diseases*, 2009, 3(2):e383.

125. Eperon G et al. Clinical presentation and treatment outcome of sleeping sickness in Sudanese pre-school children. *Acta Tropica*, 2007, 101:31–39.

126. Priotto G et al. Three drug combinations for late-stage *Trypanosoma brucei gambiense* sleeping sickness: a randomized controlled trial in Uganda. *PloS Clinical Trials*, 2006, 1(8):e39.

127. Burri C et al. Efficacy of new, concise schedule for melarsoprol in treatment of sleeping sickness caused by *Trypanosoma brucei gambiense*: a randomised trial. *The Lancet*, 2000, 355:1419–1425.

128. Pépin J et al. Short-course eflornithine in Gambian trypanosomiasis: a multicentre randomized controlled trial. *Bulletin of the World Health Organization*, 2000, 78:1284–1295.

129. Priotto G et al. Nifurtimox-eflornithine combination therapy for second-stage African *Trypanosoma brucei gambiense* trypanosomiasis: a multicentre, randomised, phase III, non-inferiority trial. *The Lancet*, 2009, 374:56–64.

130. Milord F et al. Efficacy and toxicity of eflornithine for treatment of *Trypanosoma brucei gambiense* sleeping sickness. *The Lancet*, 1992, 340:652–655.

131. Sosa Estani S et al. Efficacy of chemotherapy with benznidazole in children in the indeterminate phase of Chagas disease. *The American Journal of Tropical Medicine and Hygiene*, 1998, 59(4):526–529.

132. Andrade AL et al. Randomized trial of efficacy of benznidazole in treatment of early *Trypanosoma cruzi*. *The Lancet*, 1996, 348:1407–1413.

133. Galvão LM et al. PCR assay for monitoring *Trypanosoma cruzi* parasitemia in childhood after specific chemotherapy. *Journal of Clinical Microbiology*, 2003, 41(11):5066–5070.

134. Chippaux JP et al. Antibody drop in newborns congenitally infected by *Trypanosoma cruzi* treated with benznidazole. *Tropical Medicine and International Health*, 2010, 15(1):87–93.

135. Andrade AL et al. Short report: Benznidazole efficacy among *Trypanosoma cruzi*- infected adolescents after a six year follow up. *The American Journal of Tropical Medicine and Hygiene*, 2004, 71(5):594–587.

136. Escriba JM et al. Treatment and seroconversion in a cohort of children suffering from recent chronic Chagas infection in Yoro, Honduras. *Memórias do Instituto Oswaldo Cruz*, 2009, 104(7):986–991.

137. Yun O et al. Feasibility, drug safety, and effectiveness of etiological treatment programs for Chagas disease in Honduras, Guatemala and Bolivia: 10 year experience of Médecins sans Frontières. *PloS Neglected Tropical Diseases*, 2009, 3(7):e488.

138. Alghasham AA, Nahata MC. Clinical use of fluoroquinolones in children. *The Annals of Pharmacotherapy*, 2000, 34:347–359.

139. Yee CL et al. Tendon or joint disorders in children after treatment with fluoroquinolones or azithromycin. *The Pediatric Infectious Disease Journal*, 2002, 21(6):525–529.

140. Noel GJ et al. Comparative safety profile of levofloxacin in 2523 children with a focus on four specific musculoskeletal disorders. *The Pediatric Infectious Disease Journal*, 2007, 26:879–891.

141. Chalumeau M et al. Fluoroquinolone safety in pediatric patients: a prospective, multicenter, comparative cohort study in France. *Pediatrics*, 2003, 111:e714–e719.

142. Hunger SP, Sung L, Howard SC. Treatment strategies and regimens of graduated intensity for childhood acute lymphoblastic leukemia in low income countries: a proposal. *Pediatric Blood & Cancer*, 2009, 52(5):559–565.

143. Schrappe M, Carmitta B, Pui CH. Spotlight on long term results of pediatric ALL clinical trials from 12 study groups world wide. *Leukemia*, 2000, 14:2193–2194.

144. Patte C et al. The Société Française d'Oncologie Pédiatrique LMB89 protocol: highly effective multiagent chemotherapy tailored to the tumor burden and initial response in 561 unselected children with B-cell lymphomas and L3 leukemia. *Blood*, 2001, 7:3370–3379.

145. Hesseling PB et al. Treating Burkitt's lymphoma in Malawi, Cameroon, and Ghana. *The Lancet Oncology*, 2008, 9:512–513.

146. Uba AF, Chirdan LB. Childhood Wilms' tumour: prognostic factors in North Central Nigeria. *West African Journal of Medicine*, 2007, 26:222–225.

147. Howard S et al. Protocol-based treatment for children with cancer in low income countries in Latin America. A report on the recent meetings of the Monza International School of Pediatric Hematology/Oncology (MISPHO) Part II. *Pediatric Blood & Cancer*, 2007, 48:486–490.

148. *WHO guidelines on the pharmacological treatment of persisting pain in children with medical illnesses*. Geneva, World Health Organization, 2012.

149. Price KJ, Elliott TM. Stimulant laxatives for constipation and soiling in children. *Cochrane Database of Systematic Reviews*, 2001, (3):CD002040.

150. Myra Woolery M et al. Putting evidence into practice: evidence-based interventions for the prevention and management of constipation in patients with cancer. *Clinical Journal of Oncology Nursing*, 2008, 12 (2):317–333.

151. Freed M, Keane J, Rosenthal A. The use of heparinization to prevent arterial thrombosis after percutaneous cardiac catheterization in children. *Circulation*, 1974, 50:565–569.

152. Codispoti M et al. Individualized heparin and protamine management in infants and children undergoing cardiac operations. *The Annals of Thoracic Surgery*, 2001, 71(3):922–927.

153. Massicotte P et al. An open-label randomized controlled trial of low molecular weight heparin compared to heparin and coumadin for the treatment of venous thromboembolic events in children: the REVIVE trial. *Thrombosis Research*, 2003, 109:85–92.

154. Guzzetta N et al. A comparison of heparin management strategies in infants undergoing cardiopulmonary bypass. *Anesthesia & Analgesia*, 2008, 106(2):419–425.

155. Newall F et al. Venous thromboembolic disease: a single-centre case series study. *Journal of Paediatrics and Child Health*, 2006, 42(12):803–807.

156. Monagle P et al. Antithrombotic therapy in children. *Chest*, 2001, 119(1):344–370.

157. Massicotte P et al. An open-label randomized controlled trial of low molecular weight heparin for the prevention of central venous line-related thrombotic complications in children: the PROTEKT trial. *Thrombosis Research*, 2003, 109(2–3):101–108.

158. Hodgins S et al. Chlorhexidine gel versus aqueous for preventive use on umbilical stump. *The Pediatric Infectious Disease Journal*, 2010, 29:999–1003.

159. Mullany LC et al. Impact of umbilical cord cleansing with 4.0% chlorhexidine on time to cord separation among newborns in southern Nepal: a cluster-randomized, community-based trial. *Pediatrics*, 2006, 118:1864–1871.

160. Global maternal, newborn and child health: challenges and opportunities. (Cord Chlorhexidine Working Group, unpublished data, 2010, http://www.who.int/pmnch/events/partners_forum/3_plenary_global_mnch_bhutta_delhi_14nov.pdf, accessed 20 September 2011).

161. Mullany LC et al. Topical applications of chlorhexidine to the umbilical cord for prevention of omphalitis and neonatal mortality in southern Nepal: a community-based, cluster-randomized trial. *The Lancet*, 2006, 367(9514):910–918.

162. Gwer S et al. The role of osmotic agents in children with acute encephalopathies: a systematic review. *BMC Pediatrics*, 2010, 10:23.

163. Fiordalisi I et al. An 18-yr propective study of pediatric diabetic ketoacidosis: an approach to minimizing the risk of brain herniation during treatment. *Pediatric Diabetes*, 2007, 8(3):142–149.

164. Roberts MD et al. Diabetic ketoacidosis with intracerebral complications. *Pediatric Diabetes*, 2001, 2:109–114.

165. Brooks WA et al. Efficacy of zinc in young infants with acute watery diarrhea. *The American Journal of Clinical Nutrition*, 2005, 82(3):605–610.

166. Mazumder S et al. Effectiveness of zinc supplementation plus oral rehydration salts for diarrhoea in infants aged less than 6 months in Haryana state, India. *Bulletin of the World Health Organization*, 2010, 88(10):754–760.

167. Fischer Walker CL et al. Zinc Study Group. Zinc supplementation for the treatment of diarrhea in infants in Pakistan, India and Ethiopia. *Journal of Pediatric Gastroenterology and Nutrition*, 2006, 43(3):357–363.

168. Lazzerini M, Ronfani L. Oral zinc for treating diarrhoea in children. *Cochrane Database of Systematic Reviews*, 2008, (3):CD005436.

169. Larson CP et al. Initiation of zinc treatment for acute childhood diarrhoea, a risk for vomiting or regurgitation: a randomized double blind placebo-controlled trial. *Journal of Health, Population and Nutrition*, 2005, 23(4):311–319.

170. Bhatnagar S et al. Zinc with oral rehydration therapy reduces stool output and duration of diarrhea in hospitalized children: a randomized controlled trial. *Journal of Pediatric Gastroenterology and Nutrition*, 2004, 38(1):34–40.

171. Polat TB, Uysalol M, Çetinkaya F. Efficacy of zinc supplementation on the severity and duration of diarrhea in malnourished Turkish children. *Pediatrics International*, 2003, 45:555–559.

172. Kane MP, Abu-Baker A, Busch RS. The utility of oral diabetes medications in type 2 diabetes of the young. *Current Diabetes Reviews*, 2005, 1(1):83–92.

173. Stachnik J, Bonk ME. Inhaled anesthetic agents. *American Journal of Health-System Pharmacy*, 2006, 63:623–634.

174. Gupta A et al. Comparison of recovery profile after ambulatory anesthesia with propofol, isoflurane, sevoflurane and desflurane: a systematic review. *Anesthesia and Analgesia*, 2004, 98:632–641.

175. Lupton T, Pratt O. Intravenous drugs used for the induction of anaesthesia [Online] (http://update.anaesthesiologists.org/wp-content/uploads/2008/12/Induction-Drugs-used-in-Anaesthesia.pdf, accessed 21 September 2011).

176. Nathan N, Odin I. Induction of anaesthesia: A guide to drug choice. *Drugs*, 2007, 67:701–723.

177. Wilbur K, Zed PJ. Is propofol an optimal agent for procedural sedation and rapid sequence intubation in the emergency department? *Canadian Journal of Emergency Medicine*, 2001, 3(4):302–310.

178. Singh N et al. A comparative evaluation of oral midazolam with other sedates as premedication in pediatric dentistry. *Journal of Clinical Pediatric Dentistry*, 2002, 26(2):161–164.

179. Hunter JM. New neuromuscular blocking drugs. *New England Journal of Medicine*, 1995, 332:1691–1699.

180. Hodges SC et al. Anaesthesia in developing countries: defining the problems. *Anaesthesia*, 2007, 62:4–11.

181. Walker IA et al. Paediatric surgery and anaesthesia in south-western Uganda: a cross-sectional survey. *Bulletin of the World Health Organization*, 2010, 88:897–906.

182. Desjardins R, Ansara S, Charest J. Pre-anaesthetic medication in paediatric day-care surgery. *Canadian Anaesthetists' Society Journal*, 1981, 28(2):141–148.
183. Ong B, Ng A, Chew S. Oral premedication in paediatric day surgery. *Singapore Medical Journal* 1996, 37(2):139–142.
184. Matharu L, Ashley P. Sedation of anxious children undergoing dental treatment. *Cochrane Database of Systematic Reviews*, 2006, (1):CD003877.
185. Blanc V et al. Antiemetic prophylaxis with promethazine or droperidol in paediatric outpatient strabismus surgery. *Canadian Journal of Anesthesia*, 1991, 38(1):54–60.
186. Abu-Amara M et al. Systematic review of randomized controlled trials of pharmacological interventions to reduce ischaemia-reperfusion injury in elective liver resection with vascular occlusion. *The Official Journal of the International Hepato Pancreato Biliary Association* (Oxford), 2010, 12(1):4–14.
187. Bryson HM et al. Propofol: an update of its use in anesthesia and conscious sedation. *Drugs*, 1995, 50:513–559.
188. Hohl CM et al. Safety and clinical effectiveness of midazolam versus propofol for procedural sedation in the emergency department: a systematic review. *Academic Emergency Medicine*, 2008, 15:1–8.
189. White PF, Negus JB. Sedative infusions during local and regional anesthesia: a comparison of midazolam and propofol. *Journal of Clinical Anesthesia*, 1991, 3(1):32–39.
190. Lamond DW. Review article: safety profile of propofol for paediatric procedural sedation in the emergency department. *Emergency Medicines Australasia*, 2010, 22:265–286.
191. Migita RT et al. Sedation and analgesia for pediatric fracture reduction in the emergency department: a systematic review. *Archives of Pediatrics and Adolescent Medicine*, 2006, 160:46–51.
192. Madan R et al. Propofol as a sole agent for paediatric day care diagnostic ophthalmic procedures: comparison with halothane anaesthesia. *Paediatric Anaesthesia*, 2001, 11:671–677.
193. Wagner BK, O'Hara DA. Cost analysis of propofol versus thiopental induction anesthesia in outpatient laparoscopic gynecologic surgery. *Clinical Therapeutics*, 1995, 17(4):770–776.
194. Sung YF et al. The differential cost of anaesthesia and recovery with propofol-nitrous oxide anesthesia versus thiopental sodium-isoflurane-nitrous oxide anesthesia. *Journal of Clinical Anesthesia*, 1991, 3(5):391–394.
195. Walker KJ, Smith AF. Premedication for anxiety in adult day surgery. *Cochrane Database of Systematic Reviews*, 2009, (4):CD002192.
196. Kain ZN et al. Attenuation of the preoperative stress response with midazolam: effects on postoperative outcomes. *Anesthesiology*, 2000, 93(1):141–147.
197. Acil M et al. Perioperative effects of melatonin and midazolam premedication on sedation, orientation, anxiety scores and psychomotor performance. *European Journal of Anaesthesiology*, 2004, 21(7):553–557.
198. Fredman B et al. The effect of midazolam premedication on mental and psychomotor recovery in geriatric patients undergoing brief surgical procedures. *Anesthesia & Analgesia*, 1999, 89(5):1161–1166.
199. Naguib M, Samarkandi AH. Premedication with melatonin: a double-blind, placebo controlled comparison with midazolam. *British Journal of Anaesthesia*, 1999, 82(6):875–880.
200. Naguib M, Samarkandi AH. The comparative dose-response effects of melatonin and midazolam for premedication of adult patients: a double-blinded, placebo-controlled study. *Anesthesia & Analgesia*, 2000, 91(2):473–479.

201. Paris A et al. Effects of clonidine and midazolam premedication on bispectral index and recovery after elective surgery. *European Journal of Anaesthesiology*, 2009, 26(7):603–610.
202. Zalunardo MP et al. Quality of premedication and patient satisfaction after premedication with midazolam, clonidine or placebo : Randomized double-blind study with age-adjusted dosage. *Anaesthesist*, 2010, 59(5):410–418.
203. van Vlymen JM, Sa Rego MM, White PF. Benzodiazepine premedication: can it improve outcome in patients undergoing breast biopsy procedures? *Anesthesiology*, 1999, 90(3):740–747.
204. Hudes ET et al. A comparison of morphine-perphenazine and midazolam on preoperative sedation and arterial oxygen saturation. *Canadian Journal of Anesthesia*, 1991, 38(2):187–190.
205. Pippingskold K et al. The effect of orally administered diazepam and midazolam on plasma beta endorphin, ACTH and preoperative anxiety. *Acta Anaesthesiologica Scandinavica*, 1991, 35(2):175–180.
206. Praplan-Pahud J et al. Preoperative sedation before regional anaesthesia: comparison between zolpidem, midazolam and placebo. *British Journal of Anaesthesia*, 1990, 64(6):670–674.
207. Taittonen M et al. Cardiovascular and metabolic responses to clonidine and midazolam premedication. *European Journal of Anaesthesiology*, 1997, 14(2):190–196.
208. Kiefer RT, Weindler J, Ruprecht KW. The endocrine stress response after oral premedication with low-dose midazolam for intraocular surgery in retrobulbar anaesthesia. *European Journal of Ophthalmology*, 1998, 8(4):239–245.
209. Jalbout N et al. Premedication with midazolam (Dormicum) compared with promethazine, droperidol and placebo in relieving anxiety using Beck's anxiety inventory. *Le Journal Médical Libanais*, 1994, 42(2):69–73.
210. Aantaa R et al. A comparison of dexmedetomidine, and alpha 2-adrenoceptor agonist, and midazolam as i.m. premedication for minor gynaecological surgery. *British Journal of Anaesthesia*, 1991, 67(4):402–409.
211. Van de Velde A, Camu F, Claeys MA. Midazolam for intramuscular premedication: dose-effect relationships compared to diazepam, fentanyl and fentanyl-droperidol in a placebo controlled study. *Acta Anaesthesiologica Belgica*, 1986, 37(2):127–136.
212. Reinhart K et al. Comparison of midazolam, diazepam and placebo i.m. as premedication for regional anaesthesia. A randomized double-blind study. *British Journal of Anaesthesia*, 1985, 57(3):294–299.
213. Vinik HR, Reves JG, Wright D. Premedication with intramuscular midazolam: a prospective randomized double-blind controlled study. *Anesthesia & Analgesia*, 1982, 61(11):933–937.
214. Cox RG et al. Evidence-based clinical update: does premedication with oral midazolam lead to improved behavioural outcomes in children? *Canadian Journal of Anesthesia*, 2006, 53(12):1213–1219.
215. Hosey MT et al. The effect of transmucosal 0.2 mg/kg midazolam premedication on dental anxiety, anaesthetic induction and psychological morbidity in children undergoing general anaesthesia for tooth extraction. *British Dental Journal*, 2009, 207(E2):32–33.
216. Isik B, Baygin O, Bodur H. Premedication with melatonin vs midazolam in anxious children. *Paediatric Anaesthesia*, 2008, 18(7):635–641.
217. Finley GA et al. High levels of impulsivity may contraindicate midazolam premedication in children. *Canadian Journal of Anesthesia*, 2006, 53(1):73–78.
218. Mishra LD et al. Injectable midazolam as oral premedicant in pediatric neurosurgery. *Journal of Neurosurgical Anesthesiology*, 2005, 17(4):193–198.

219. Samarkandi A et al. Melatonin vs. midazolam premedication in children: a double-blind, placebo controlled study. *European Journal of Anaesthesiology*, 2005, 22(3):189–196.

220. Howell TK et al. A comparison of oral transmucosal fentanyl and oral midazolam for premedication in children. *Anaesthesia*, 2002, 57(8):798–805.

221. Pandit UA et al. Oral transmucosal midazolam premedication for preschool children. *Canadian Journal of Anesthesia*, 2001, 48(2):191–195.

222. Fazi L et al. A comparison of oral clonidine and oral midazolam as preanesthetic medications in the pediatric tonsillectomy patient. *Anesthesia & Analgesia*, 2001, 92(1):56–61.

223. Khalil S et al. Sublingual midazolam premedication in children: a dose response study. *Paediatric Anaesthesia*, 1998, 8(6):461–465.

224. McGraw T, Kendrick A. Oral midazolam premedication and postoperative behaviour in children. *Paediatric Anaesthesia*, 1998, 8(2):117–121.

225. Riva J et al. Oral premedication with midazolam in paediatric anaesthesia. Effects on sedation and gastric contents. *Paediatric Anaesthesia*, 1997, 7(3):191–196.

226. Gillerman RG et al. Parental presence plus oral midazolam decreases frequency of 5% halothane inductions in children. *Journal of Clinical Anesthesia*, 1996, 8(6):480–485.

227. Cray SH et al. Oral midazolam premedication for paediatric day case patients. *Paediatric Anaesthesia*, 1996, 6(4):265–270.

228. McMillan CO et al. Premedication of children with oral midazolam. *Canadian Journal of Anesthesia*, 1992, 39(6):545–550.

229. Roelofse JA, van der Bijl P. Comparison of rectal midazolam and diazepam for premedication in pediatric dental patients. *Journal of Oral and Maxillofacial Surgery*, 1993, 51(5):525–529.

230. Roelofse JA et al. Preanesthetic medication with rectal midazolam in children undergoing dental extractions. *Journal of Oral and Maxillofacial Surgery*, 1990, 48(8):791–797.

231. Vetter TR. A comparison of midazolam, diazepam, and placebo as oral anesthetic premedicants in younger children. *Journal of Clinical Anesthesia*, 1993, 5(1):58–61.

232. Gallardo F et al. Oral midazolam as premedication for the apprehensive child before dental treatment. *Journal of Clinical Pediatric Dentistry*, 1994, 18(2):123–127.

233. Liacouras CA et al. Placebo-controlled trial assessing the use of oral midazolam as a premedication to conscious sedation for pediatric endoscopy. *Gastrointestinal Endoscopy*, 1998, 47(6):455–460.

234. Bevan JC et al. Midazolam premedication delays recovery after propofol without modifying involuntary movements. *Anesthesia & Analgesia*, 1997, 85(1):50–54.

235. Viitanen H et al. Premedication with midazolam delays recovery after ambulatory sevoflurane anesthesia in children. *Anesthesia & Analgesia*, 1999, 89(1):75–79.

236. Viitanen H et al. Midazolam premedication delays recovery from propofol-induced sevoflurane anesthesia in children 1-3 yr. *Canadian Journal of Anesthesia*, 1999, 46(8):766–771.

237. Riad W et al. Effect of midazolam, dexamethasone and their combination on the prevention of nausea and vomiting following strabismus repair in children. *European Journal of Anaesthesiology*, 2007, 24(8):697–701.

238. Splinter WM et al. Midazolam reduces vomiting after tonsillectomy in children. *Canadian Journal of Anesthesia*, 1995, 42(3):201–203.

239. McQuaid KR, Laine L. A systematic review and meta-analysis of randomized, controlled trials of moderate sedation for routine endoscopic procedures. *Gastrointestinal Endoscopy*, 2008, 67(6):910–923.

240. Stewart SH et al. Effects of midazolam on explicit vs implicit memory in a pediatric surgery setting. *Psychopharmacology (Berl)*, 2006, 188(4):489–497.
241. Wan K, Jing Q, Zhao JZ. Evaluation of oral midazolam as conscious sedation for pediatric patients in oral restoration. *Chinese Medical Sciences Journal*, 2006, 21(3):163–166.
242. Herd DW et al. Conscious sedation reduces distress in children undergoing voiding cystourethrography and does not interfere with the diagnosis of vesicoureteric reflux: a randomized controlled study. *American Journal of Roentgenology*, 2006, 187(6):1621–1626.
243. Stokland E et al. Sedation with midazolam for voiding cystourethrography in children: a randomized double-blind study. *Pediatric Radiology*, 2003, 33(4):247–249.
244. Shane SA, Fuchs SM, Khine H. Efficacy of rectal midazolam for the sedation of preschool children undergoing laceration repair. *Annals of Emergency Medicine*, 1994, 24(6):1065–1073.
245. Theroux MC et al. Efficacy of intranasal midazolam in facilitating suturing of lacerations in preschool children in the emergency department. *Pediatrics*, 1993, 91(3):624–627.
246. Hennes HM et al. The effect of oral midazolam on anxiety of preschool children during laceration repair. *Annals of Emergency Medicine*, 1990, 19(9):1006–1009.
247. Golparvar M et al. Paradoxical reaction following intravenous midazolam premedication in pediatric patients - a randomized placebo controlled trial of ketamine for rapid tranquilization. *Paediatric Anaesthesia*, 2004, 14(11):924–930.
248. Brok J, Buckely N, Gluud C. Interventions for paracetamol (acetaminophen) overdose. *Cochrane Database of Systematic Reviews*, 2006, (2):CD003328.
249. Crump JA et al. The global burden of typhoid fever. *Bulletin of the World Health Organization*, 2004, 82:346.
250. Arjyal et al. Gatifloxacin versus chloramphenicol: an open, randomized controlled treatment of uncomplicated enteric fever. *The Lancet Infectious Diseases*, 2011, 11(6):445–454.
251. Dolecek C et al. A multi-centre randomized controlled trial of gatifloxacin versus azithromycin for the treatment of uncomplicated typhoid and paratyphoid fever in children and adults in Vietnam. *PLoS ONE*, 2008, 3(5):e2188.
252. Pandit A et al. An open randomized comparison of gatifloxacin versus cefixime for the treatment of uncomplicated enteric fever. *PLoS ONE*, 2007, 2(6):e542.
253. Pichichero ME et al. Safety and efficacy of gatifloxacin therapy for children with recurrent acute otitis media (AOM) and/or AOM treatment failure. *Clinical Infectious Diseases*, 2005, 41:470.
254. Katlama C et al. Efficacy and safety of etravirine in treatment-experienced, HIV-1 patients: pooled 48 week analysis of two randomized, controlled trials. *AIDS*, 2009, 23(17):2289–2300.
255. Fullerton DS et al. Pharmacoeconomics of etravirine. *Pharmacoeconomics Outcomes Research*, 2010, 10(5):485–495.
256. Clotet B et al. Efficacy and safety of darunavir-ritonavir at week 48 in treatment-experienced patients with HIV-1 infection in POWER 1 and 2: a pooled subgroup analysis of data from two randomized trials. *The Lancet*, 2007, 369(9568):1169–1178.
257. Madruga JV et al. Efficacy and safety of darunavir-ritonavir compared with that of lopinavir-ritonavir at 48 weeks in treatment-experienced, HIV-infected patients in TITAN: a randomized controlled phase III trial. *The Lancet*, 2007, 370(9581):49–58.
258. Banhegyi D et al. *Phase III TITAN Week 96 final analysis: efficacy/safety of darunavir/ritonavir versus lopinavir/ritonavir in lopinavir/ritonavir-naïve, treatment-experienced patients*. Presented at the 9th International Congress on HIV and Drug Therapy in HIV Infection, Glasgow, 2008 (http://www.tibotec.com/content/congresses/www.tibotec.com/Banhegyi_TMC114_TITAN_96w.pdf, accessed 21 September 2011).

259. Molina JM et al. Safety and efficacy of darunavir (TMC114) with low-dose ritonavir in treatment-experienced patients: 24-week results of POWER 3. *Journal of Acquired Immune Deficiency Syndromes*, 2007, 46(1):24–31.

260. Blanche S et al. Pharmacokinetics, safety and efficacy of darunavir/ritonavir in treatment-experienced children and adolescents. *AIDS*, 2009, 23(15):2005–2013.

261. Mauskopf J et al. A review of economic evaluations of darunavir boosted by low-dose ritonavir in treatment-experienced persons living with HIV infection. *Pharmacoeconomics*, 2010, 28(Suppl. 1):1–16.

262. Grinsztejn B et al. Safety and efficacy of the HIV-1 integrase inhibitor raltegravir (MK-0518) in treatment-experienced patients with multidrug-resistant virus: a phase II randomized controlled trial. *The Lancet*, 2007, 369(9569):1261–1269.

263. Steigbigel RT et al. Raltegravir with optimized background therapy for resistant HIV-1 infection. *The New England Journal of Medicine*, 2008, 359(4):339–354.

264. Gatell JM et al. Long-term efficacy and safety of the HIV integrase inhibitor raltegravir in patients with limited treatment options in a Phase II study. *Journal of Acquired Immune Deficiency Syndromes*, 2010, 53(4):456–463.

265. Steigbigel RT et al. Long-term efficacy and safety of raltegravir combined with optimized background therapy in treatment-experienced patients with drug-resistant HIV infection: week 96 results of the BENCHMARK 1 and 2 Phase III trials. *Clinical Infectious Diseases*, 2010, 50(4):605–612.

266. Sundar S et al. Comparison of short-course multidrug treatment with standard therapy for visceral leishmaniasis in India: an open-label, non-inferiority, randomised controlled trial. *The Lancet*, 2011, 377(9764):477–486.

267. Sirima SB et al. The efficacy and safety of a new fixed-dose combination of amodiaquine and artesunate in young African children with acute uncomplicated *Plasmodium falciparum*. *Malaria Journal*, 2009, 8:48.

268. Ndiyae JL et al. Randomized multicentre assessment of the efficacy and safety of ASAQ – a fixed-dose artesunate-amodiaquine combination therapy in the treatment of uncomplicated *Plasmodium falciparum* malaria. *Malaria Journal*, 2009, 8:125.

269. Sinclair D et al. Artemisinin-based combination therapy for treating uncomplicated malaria. *Cochrane Database of Systematic Reviews*, 2009, (3):CD007483.

270. Tshefu AK et al. Efficacy and safety of a fixed-dose oral combination of pyronaridine-artesunate compared with artemether-lumefantrine in children and adults with uncomplicated *Plasmodium falciparum* malaria: a randomized non-inferiority trial. *The Lancet*, 2010, 375:1457–1467.

271. Poravuth Y et al. Pyronaridine-artesunate versus chloroquine in patients with acute *Plasmodium vivax* malaria. *PLoS ONE*, 2011, 6(1):e14501.

272. Ghersi D et al. Taxane containing regimens for metastatic breast cancer. *Cochrane Database of Systematic Reviews*, 2005, (2): CD003366.

273. De Laurentiis M et al. Taxane-based combinations as adjuvant chemotherapy for early breast cancer: a meta-analysis of randomized trials. *Journal of Clinical Oncolology*, 2008, 26:44–56.

274. Ferguson T et al. Taxanes for adjuvant treatment of early breast cancer. *Cochrane Database of Systematic Reviews*, 2007, (4): CD004421.

275. *Guidance on the use of paclitaxel in the treatment of ovarian cancer*. Technology Appraisal No. 55. London, National Institute for Health and Clinical Excellence, 2003 (http://www.nice.org.uk/nicemedia/live/11486/32539/32539.pdf, accessed 21 September 2011).

276. CRASH-2 trial collaborators. Effects of tranexamic acid on death, vascular occlusive events, and blood transfusion in trauma patients with significant haemorrhage (CRASH-2): a randomised placebo controlled trial. *The Lancet*, 2010, 376(9734):23–32.
277. *Chronic heart failure: management of chronic heart failure in adults in primary and secondary care*. Full guidelines. London, National Institute for Health and Clinical Excellence, 2010 (http://www.nice.org.uk/CG108, accessed 21 September 2011).
278. HFSA. Heart Failure Society of America 2010 comprehensive heart failure practice guideline. *Journal of Cardiac Failure*, 2010, 16(6):e1–194.
279. CIBIS II investigators and committees. The cardiac insufficiency bisoprolol study II (CIBIS II): a randomised trial. *The Lancet*, 1999, 353:9–13.
280. MERIT-HF Study Group. Effect of metoprolol CR/XL in chronic heart failure: Metoprolol CR/XL randomised intervention trial in congestive heart failure (MERIT-HF). *The Lancet*, 1999, 353:2001–2009.
281. Eichhorn EJ, Bristow MR. Commentary: the carvedilol prospective randomized cumulative survival (COPERNICUS) trail. *Current Controlled Trials in Cardiovascular Medicine*, 2001, 2:20–23.
282. Funck-Brentano C. Beta-blockade in CHF: from contraindication to indication. *European Heart Journal Supplements*, 2006, 8(Suppl. C) :C19–C27.
283. Bangalore S et al. Cardiovascular protecting using beta-blockers: a critical review of the evidence. *Journal of the American College of Cardiology*, 2007, 50:563–572.
284. Shibata MC et al. Systematic review of the impact of beta-blockers on mortality and hospital admissions in heart failure. *European Journal of Heart Failure*, 2001, 3(3):351–357.
285. Dulin BR et al. Do elderly systolic heart failure patients benefit from beta-blockers to the same extent as the non-elderly? Meta-analysis of 12,000 patients in large-scale clinical trials. *American Journal of Cardiology*, 2005, 95:896–898.
286. Haas SJ et al. Are beta-blockers as efficacious in patients with diabetes mellitus as in patients without diabetes mellitus who have chronic heart failure? A meta-analysis of large-scale clinical trials. *American Heart Journal*, 2003, 146:848–853.
287. Bouzamondo A et al. Beta-blocker benefit according to severity of heart failure. *European Journal of Heart Failure*, 2003, 5:281–289.
288. Krum H et al. Prognostic benefit of beta-blockers in patients not receiving ACE-inhibitors. *European Heart Journal*, 2005, 26:2154–2158.
289. Salpeter SS et al. Cardioselective beta-blockers for chronic obstructive pulmonary disease. *Cochrane Database of Systematic Reviews*, 2005, (4):CD003566.
290. Gibbons RJ et al. ACC/AHA 2002 guideline update for the management of patients with chronic stable angina. *Journal of the American College of Cardiology*, 2003, 41:159–168.
291. Weber F et al. Prognostic implications of autonomic function assessed by analyses of catecholamines and heart rate variability in stable angina pectoris. *European Heart Journal*, 1999, 20:38–50.
292. Konishi M et al. Comparative effects of carvedilol vs bisoprolol for severe congestive heart failure. *Circulation Journal*, 2010, 74(6):1127–1134.
293. Ishiguro H et al. Antiarrhythmic effect of bisoprolol, a highly selective ß1-blocker in patients with paroxysmal atrial fibrillation. *International Heart Journal*, 2008, 49(3):281–293.
294. Plewan A et al. Maintenance of sinus rhythm after electrical cardioversion of persistent atrial fibrillation: sotalol vs bisoprolol. *European Heart Journal*, 2001, 22(16):1504–1510.

295. Hiltunen TP et al. Predictors of antihypertensive drug responses: initial data from a placebo-controlled, randomized, cross-over study with four antihypertensive drugs (The GENRES Study). *American Journal of Hypertension*, 2007, 20(3):311–318.

296. Neutel JM et al. Application of ambulatory blood pressure monitoring in differentiating between antihypertensive agents. *American Journal of Medicine*, 1993, 94:181–187.

297. Deary AJ et al. Double blind, placebo controlled crossover comparison of five classes of antihypertensive drugs. *Journal of Hypertension*, 2002, 20:771–777.

298. Carlberg B et al. Atenolol in hypertension: is it a wise choice? *The Lancet*, 2004, 364(9446): 1684–1689.

299. Koning S et al. Interventions for impetigo. *Cochrane Database of Systematic Reviews*, 2003, (2):CD003261.

300. Bergfeld WF et al. Safety assessment of basic violet 1, basic violet 3 and basic violet 4. *International Journal of Toxicology*, 2009, 28(Suppl. 2):S193–S204.

301. Au W et al. Further study of the genetic toxicity of gentian violet. *Mutation Research*, 1979, 66:103–112.

302. Diaz M et al. Efficacy, safety and acceptability of precipitated sulphur petrolatum for topical treatment of scabies at the city of Coro, Falcon State, Venezuela. *Revista de Investigación Clínica*, 2004, 56:615–622.

303. Singalavanija S et al. A comparative study between 10 per cent sulfur ointment and 0.3 per cent gamma benzene hexachloride gel in the treatment of scabies in children. *Journal of the Medical Association of Thailand*, 2003, 86(Suppl. 3):S531–S536.

304. Moayyedi P et al. Pharmacological interventions for non-ulcer dyspepsia. *Cochrane Database of Systematic Reviews*, 2006, (4):CD001960.

305. Ford AC et al. Eradication therapy for peptic ulcer disease in *Helicobacter pylori* positive patients. *Cochrane Database of Systematic Reviews*, 2003, (4):CD003840.

306. Kiltz U et al. Use of NSAIDs and infection with *Helicobacter pylori*–what does the rheumatologist need to know? *Rheumatology* (Oxford), 2008, 47(9):1342–1347.

307. Gisbert JP et al. *Helicobacter pylori* eradication therapy vs. antisecretory non-eradication therapy (with or without long-term maintenance antisecretory therapy) for the prevention of recurrent bleeding from peptic ulcer. *Cochrane Database of Systematic Reviews*, 2004, (2):CD004062.

308. Yaghoobi M et al. Is there an increased risk of GERD after *Helicobacter pylori* eradication? A meta-analysis. *American Journal of Gastroenterology*, 2010, 105(5):1007–1013.

309. Chey WD, Wong BCY, and the Practice Parameters Committee of the American College of Gastroenterology. American College of Gastroenterology guideline on the management of *Helicobacter pylori* infection. *American Journal of Gastroenterology*, 2007, 102:1808–1825.

310. Malfertheiner P et al. The European Helicobacter Study Group (EHSG). Current concepts in the management of *Helicobacter pylori* infection: the Maastricht III consensus report. *GUT*, 2007, 56:772–781.

311. Fuccio L et al. Meta-analysis: duration of first-line proton-pump inhibitor based triple therapy for *Helicobacter pylori* eradication. *Annals of Internal Medicine*, 2007, 147:553–562.

312. Kim SY et al. Comparative study of *Helicobacter pylori* eradication rates of twice- versus four-times-daily amoxicillin administered with proton pump inhibitor and clarithromycin: a randomized study. *Helicobacter*, 2008, 13(4):282–287.

313. Ben Mansour K et al. Primary resistance to clarithromycin, metronidazole and amoxicillin of *Helicobacter pylori* isolated from Tunisian patients with peptic ulcers and gastritis: a prospective multicentre study. *Annals of Clinical Microbiology and Antimicrobials*, 2010, 9(1):22.
314. Taylor JL et al. Pharmacoeconomic comparison of treatments for the eradication of *Helicobacter pylori*. *Archives of Internal Medicine*, 1997, 157(1):87–97.
315. Sancar M et al. Pharmacoeconomic comparison of *Helicobacter pylori* eradication regimens. *Pharmacy World and Science*, 2006, 28(4):207–214.
316. Uygun A et al. The efficacy of bismuth containing quadruple therapy as a first-line treatment option for *Helicobacter pylori*. *Journal of Digestive Diseases*, 2007, 8(4):211–215.
317. Palmer KR et al. Double-blind cross-over study comparing loperamide, codeine and diphenoxylate in the treatment of chronic diarrhoea. *Gastroenterology*, 1980, 79:1272–1275.
318. Van Loon FP et al. Double blind trial of loperamide for treating acute watery diarrhoea in expatriates in Bangladesh. *GUT*, 1989, 30:492–495.
319. Barbezat GO et al. A double-blind trial of loperamide in the treatment of chronic diarrhoea. *South African Medical Journal*, 1979, 55(13):502–503.
320. Allison MC et al. A double-blind crossover comparison of limidine, loperamide and placebo for the control of chronic diarrhoea. *Alimentary Pharmacology and Therapeutics*, 1988, 2:347–351.
321. Bergström T et al. Symptomatic treatment of acute infectious diarrhoea: loperamide versus placebo in a double-blind trial. *Journal of Infection*, 1985, 12:35–38.
322. Cascinu S et al. Octreotide versus loperamide in the treatment of fluorouracil-induced diarrhea: a randomized trial. *Journal of Clinical Oncology*, 1993, 11(1):148–151.
323. Gebbia V et al. Subcutaneous octreotide versus oral loperamide in the treatment of diarrhea following chemotherapy. *Anti-Cancer Drugs*, 1993, 4:443–445.
324. Dupont HL et al. Comparative efficacy of loperamide hydrochloride and bismuth subsalicylate in the management of acute diarrhea. *American Journal of Medicine*, 1990, 88(6A):15S–19S.
325. Johnson PC et al. Comparison of loperamide with bismuth subsalicylate for the treatment of acute travellers' diarrhea. *Journal of the American Medical Association*, 1986, 255(6):757–760.
326. Dupont HL et al. A randomized, open-label comparison of nonprescription loperamide and attapulgite in the symptomatic treatment of acute diarrhea. *American Journal of Medicine*, 1990, 88(6A):20S–23S.
327. Wang HH et al. A blind, randomized comparison of racecadotril and loperamide for stopping acute diarrhoea in adults. *World Journal of Gastroenterology*, 2005, 11(10):1540–1543.
328. Gallelli L et al. Prospective randomized double-blind trial of racecadotril compared with loperamide in elderly people with gastroenteritis living in nursing homes. *The Journal of Clinical Pharmacology*, 2009, 66:137–144.
329. Vetel JM et al. Comparison of racecadotril and loperamide in adults with acute diarrhoea. *Alimentary Pharmacology and Therapeutics*, 1999, 13(Suppl. 6):S21–S26.
330. Prado D (for the Global Adult Racecadotril Study Group). A multinational comparison of racecadotril and loperamide in the treatment of acute watery diarrhoea in adults. *Scandinavian Journal of Gastroenterology*, 2002, 6:656–661.
331. Kaplan MA et al. Loperamide-simethicone vs loperamide alone, simethicone alone and placebo in the treatment of acute diarrhea with gas-related abdominal discomfort. *Archives of Family Medicine*, 1999, 8:243–248.

332. Hanauer SB et al. Randomized, double blind, placebo-controlled clinical trial of loperamide plus simethicone versus loperamide alone and simethicone alone in the treatment of acute diarrhea with gas-related abdominal discomfort. *Current Medical Research and Opinion*, 2007, 23(5):1033–1043.

333. Mainguet P, Fiasse R. Double-blind placebo-controlled study of loperamide (Imodium) in chronic diarrhoea caused by iliocolic disease or resection. *GUT*, 1977, 18:575–579.

334. Doren M, Nilsson JA, Johnell O. Effects of specific post-menopausal hormone therapies on bone mineral density in post-menopausal women: a meta-analysis. *Human Reproduction*, 2003, 18(8):1737–1746.

335. Million Women Study Collaborators. Breast cancer and hormone-replacement therapy in the Million Women Study. *The Lancet*, 2003, 362:429–437.

336. Gabriel SR et al. Hormone replacement therapy for preventing cardiovascular disease in post-menopausal women. *Cochrane Database of Systematic Reviews*, 2005, (2): CD002229.

337. Waters DD et al. Effects of hormone replacement therapy and antioxidant vitamin supplements on coronary atherosclerosis in postmenopausal women. A randomized controlled trial. *Journal of the American Medical Association*, 2002, 288:2432–2440.

338. Pal D et al. Neonatal hypoglycaemia in Nepal 1. Prevalence and risk factors. *Archives of Disease in Childhood, Fetal and Neonatal Edition*, 2000, 82:F46–F51.

339. Güven M et al. Evaluation of patients admitted with hypoglycaemia to a teaching hospital in Central Anatolia. *Postgraduate Medical Journal*, 2000, 76:150–152.

340. Bassili A et al. The adequacy of diabetic care for children in a developing country. *Diabetes Research and Clinical Practice*, 2001, 53:187–199.

341. Wexler DJ et al. Prevalence of hyper- and hypoglycemia among inpatients with diabetes. *Diabetes Care*, 2007, 30(2):367–369.

342. Elusiyan JBE et al. Hypoglycaemia in a Nigerian paediatric emergency ward. *Journal of Tropical Pediatrics*, 2005, 52:96–102.

343. Osier FH et al. Abnormal blood glucose concentrations on admission to a rural Kenyan district hospital: prevalence and outcome. *Archives of Disease in Childhood*, 2003, 88:621–625.

344. Solomon T et al. Hypoglycaemia in paediatric admissions in Mozambique. *The Lancet*, 1994, 343:149–150.

345. Mühlhauser I, Koch J, Berger M. Pharmacokinetics and bioavailability of injected glucagon. *Diabetes Care*, 1985:39–42.

346. Casparie AE, Elving LD. Severe hypoglycemia in diabetic patients: frequency, causes, prevention. *Diabetes Care*, 1983, 8:141–145.

347. Collier A et al. Comparison of intravenous glucagon and dextrose in treatment of severe hypoglycemia in an accident and emergency department. *Diabetes Care*, 1987, 10:712–714.

348. Singh SR et al. Efficacy and safety of insulin analogues for the management of diabetes mellitus: A meta-analysis. *Canadian Medical Association Journal*, 2009, 180(4):385–397.

349. *WHO Recommendations for the prevention of postpartum haemorrhage*. Geneva, World Health Organization, 2007.

350. *WHO guidelines for the management of postpartum haemorrhage and retained placenta*. Geneva, World Health Organization, 2009.

351. ICM, FIGO. *Prevention and treatment of post-partum haemorrhage: new advances for low resource settings. A joint statement*. The Hague, International Confederation of Midwives; London, International Federation of Gynecology and Obstetrics, 2003.

352. Royal College of Obstetricians and Gynaecologists. *RCOG green-top Guideline no. 52*. London, 2009.

353. American College of Obstetricians and Gynecologists. ACOG practice bulletin no. 76. Postpartum hemorrhage. *Obstetrics & Gynecology*, 2006, 108:1039–1047.

354. Walraven G et al. Management of post-partum hemorrhage in low-income countries. *Best Practice & Research Clinical Obstetrics and Gynecology*, 2008, 22(6):1013–1023.

355. Høj L et al. Effect of sublingual misoprostol on severe postpartum hemorrhage in a primary health centre in Guinea-Bissau: randomised double blind clinical trial. *British Medical Journal*, 2005, 331(7519):723.

356. Derman RJ et al. Oral misoprostol in preventing postpartum haemorrhage in resource-poor communities: a randomised controlled trial. *The Lancet*, 2006, 368:1248–1253.

357. Mobeen N et al. Administration of misoprostol by trained traditional birth attendants to prevent postpartum haemorrhage in homebirths in Pakistan: a randomised placebo-controlled trial. *British Journal of Obstetrics and Gynaecology*, 2011, 118(3):353–361.

358. Blum J et al. Treatment of postpartum hemorrhage with misoprostol. *International Journal of Gynecology & Obstetrics*, 2007, 99:S202–S205.

359. Winikoff B et al. Treatment of post-partum haemorrhage with sublingual misoprostol versus oxytocin in women not exposed to oxytocin during labour: a double-blind randomised non-inferiority trial. *The Lancet*, 2010, 375(9710):210–216.

360. Lumbiganon P et al. Misoprostol dose–related shivering and pyrexia in the third stage of labour. *British Journal of Obstetrics and Gynaecology*, 1999, 106:304–308.

361. Khan RU, El-Rafaey H. Pharmacokinetics and adverse-effect profile of rectally administered misoprostol in the third stage of labor. *Obstetrics & Gynecology*, 2003, 101:968–974.

362. Hofmeyr GJ et al. Misoprostol to prevent and treat postpartum haemorrhage: a systematic review and meta-analysis of maternal deaths and dose-related effects. *Bulletin of the World Health Organization*, 2009, 87(9):666–677.

363. Gülmezoglu AM et al. Prostaglandins for preventing postpartum haemorrhage. *Cochrane Database of Systematic Reviews*, 2007, (3):CD000494.

364. Hofmeyr GJ, Gülmezoglu AM. Misoprostol for the prevention and treatment of postpartum haemorrhage. *Best Practice & Research Clinical Obstetrics and Gynaecology*, 2008, 22(6):1025–1041.

365. Blum J et al. Treatment of post-partum haemorrhage with sublingual misoprostol versus oxytocin in women receiving prophylactic oxytocin: a double-blind, randomised, non-inferiority trial. *The Lancet*, 2010, 375(9710):217–223.

366. Strand RT et al. Postpartum hemorrhage: a prospective, comparative study in Angola using a new disposable device for oxytocin administration. *Acta Obstetricia et Gynecologica Scandinavica*, 2005, 84:260–265.

367. Reproductive Health Department (Ministry of Health) Viet Nam, PATH. *Reducing postpartum hemorrhage in Thanh Hoa, Viet Nam: Assessing the role of active management of third stage of labor and of oxytocin in ampoules and Uniject devices*. Research report. Seattle, Program for Appropriate Technology in Health, 2005.

368. Tsu VD et al. Oxytocin in prefilled Uniject injection devices for managing third-stage labor in Indonesia. *International Journal of Gynaecology and Obstetrics*, 2003, 83(1):103–111.

369. PATH. *Technology solutions for global health: oxytocin in Uniject*. Seattle, Program for Appropriate Technology in Health, 2010 (http://www.path.org/files/TS_update_uniject_oxytocin.pdf, accessed 26 January 2011).

370. Simmonsen L et al. Unsafe injections in the developing world and transmission of bloodborne pathogens: a review. *Bulletin of the World Health Organization*, 1999, 77:801–807.

371. Gisselquist D et al. HIV infections in sub-Saharan Africa not explained by sexual or vertical transmission. *International Journal of STD and AIDS*, 2002, 13:657–666.

372. *Global strategy for the diagnosis and management of asthma in children 5 years and younger.* Global Initiative for Asthma, 2009 (http://www.ginasthma.org/guidelines-gina-report-global-strategy-for-asthma.html, accessed 30 September 2011).

373. *GINA report, global strategy for asthma management and prevention*. Global Initiative for Asthma, 2010 (http://www.ginasthma.org/guidelines-gina-report-global-strategy-for-asthma.html, accessed 30 September 2011).

374. The British Thoracic Society and the Scottish Intercollegiate Guidelines Network. *British guideline on the management of asthma: quick reference guide*. United Kingdom, 2008.

375. American National Heart, Lung, and Blood Institute, National Asthma Education and Prevention Program. *Expert Panel Report 3: guidelines for the diagnosis and management of asthma full report*, 2007. (http://www.nhlbi.nih.gov/guidelines/asthma/asthgdln.pdf, accessed 29 September 2011).

376. *Electronic therapeutic guidelines*. Australia, 2009, Version 4 (http://www.tg.org.au/index.php?sectionid=49, accessed 21 September 2011).

377. Rai SP et al. Best treatment guidelines for bronchial asthma (India). *Medical Journal Armed Forces India*, 2007, 63(3): 264–268.

378. *Management of asthma – guidelines*. Sri Lanka Medical Association, 2006.

379. *National best management guidelines – bronchial asthma*. Sri Lanka College of Paediatricians, 2007.

380. *WHO Pocket book of hospital care for children: guidelines for the management of common illnesses with limited resources*. Geneva, World Health Organization, 2005 (http://whqlibdoc.who.int/publications/2005/9241546700.pdf, accessed 30 September 2011).

381. Gupta P et al. Oral salbutamol for symptomatic relief in mild bronchiolitis: a double blind randomized placebo-controlled trial. *Indian Pediatrics*, 2008, 45(7):547–553.

382. Patel H, Gouin S, Platt RW. Randomized, double-blind, placebo-controlled trial of oral albuterol in infants with mild-to-moderate acute viral bronchiolitis. *Journal of Pediatrics*, 2003, 142(5):509–514.

383. Cengizlier R et al. Effect of oral and inhaled salbutamol in infants with bronchiolitis. *Acta Paediatrica Japonica*, 1997, 39(1):61–63.

384. Gadomski AM, Bhasale AL. Bronchodilators for bronchiolitis. *Cochrane Database of Systematic Reviews*, 2006, (3):CD001266.

385. Smucny J, Becker LA, Glazier R. Beta2-agonists for acute bronchitis. *Cochrane Database of Systematic Reviews*, 2006, (4):CD001726.

386. Scottish Intercollegiates Guidelines Network (SIGN). *Bronchiolitis in children — a national clinical guideline*. NHS Quality Improvement Scotland, 2006.

387. Robertson J et al. What essential medicines for children are on the shelf? *Bulletin of the World Health Organization*, 2009, 87(3):231–237.

388. Kotwani A. Availability, price and affordability of asthma medicines in five Indian states. *The International Journal of Tuberculosis and Lung Disease*, 2009, 13(5):574–579.

389. Steinberg MH et al. Effect of hydroxyurea on mortality and morbidity in adult sickle cell anemia. Risks and benefits up to 9 years of treatment. *Journal of the American Medical Association*, 2003, 289:1645–1651.

390. Saad ST et al. Follow-up of sickle cell disease patients with priapism treated by hydroxyurea. *American Journal of Hematology*, 2004, 77:45–49.
391. Strouse JJ et al. Hydroxyurea for sickle cell disease: a systematic review for efficacy and toxicity in children. *Pediatrics*, 2008, 122:1332–1342.
392. Gaston MH et al. Prophylaxis with oral penicillin in children with sickle cell anemia. A randomized trial. *The New England Journal of Medicine*, 1986, 314:1593–1599.
393. Dominguez-Cherit G et al. Critically ill patients with 2009 influenza A(H1N1) in Mexico. *Journal of the American Medical Association*, 2009, 302(17):1880–1887.
394. Echevarria-Zuno S et al. Infection and death from influenza A H1N1 virus in Mexico: a retrospective analysis. *The Lancet*, 2009, 374(9707):2072–2079.
395. Jain S et al. Hospitalized patients with 2009 H1N1 influenza in the United States, April-June 2009. *The New England Journal of Medicine*, 2009, 361(20):1935–1944.
396. Jamieson DJ et al. H1N1 2009 influenza virus infection during pregnancy in the USA. *The Lancet*, 2009, 374(9688):451–458.
397. Louie JK et al. Factors associated with death or hospitalization due to pandemic 2009 influenza A(H1N1) infection in California. *Journal of the American Medical Association*, 2009, 302(17):1896–1902.
398. Shun-Shin M et al. Neuraminidase inhibitors for treatment and prophylaxis of influenza in children: systematic review and meta-analysis of randomised controlled trials. *British Medical Journal*, 2009, 339:b3172.
399. Kaiser L et al. Impact of oseltamivir treatment on influenza-related lower respiratory tract complications and hospitalizations. *Archives of Internal Medicine*, 2003, 163(14):1667–1672.
400. Jefferson T et al. Neuraminidase inhibitors for preventing and treating influenza in healthy adults: systematic review and meta-analysis. *British Medical Journal*, 2009, 339:b5106.
401. Freemantle N, Calvert M. What can we learn from observational studies of oseltamivir to treat influenza in healthy adults? *British Medical Journal*, 2009, 339:b5248.
402. Doshi P. Neuraminidase inhibitors — the story behind the Cochrane Review. *British Medical Journal*, 2009, 339:b5164.
403. Godlee F, Clarke M. Why don't we have all the evidence on oseltamivir? *British Medical Journal*, 2009, 339:b5351.
404. Hanshaoworakul W et al. Severe human influenza infections in Thailand: oseltamivir treatment and risk factors for fatal outcome. *PLoS ONE*, 2009, 4(6):e6051.
405. Casscells SW et al. Use of oseltamivir after influenza infection is associated with reduced incidence of recurrent adverse cardiovascular outcomes among military health system beneficiaries with prior cardiovascular diseases. *Circulation: Cardiovascular Quality and Outcomes*, 2009, 2(2):108–115.
406. Piedra PA, Schulman KL, Blumentals WA. Effects of oseltamivir on influenza-related complications in children with chronic medical conditions. *Pediatrics*, 2009, 124(1):170–178.
407. Barr CE et al. Effect of oseltamivir on the risk of pneumonia and use of health care services in children with clinically diagnosed influenza. *Current Medical Research and Opinion*, 2007, 23(3):523–531.
408. Bowles SK et al. Use of oseltamivir during influenza outbreaks in Ontario nursing homes, 1999-2000. *Journal of the American Geriatrics Society*, 2002, 50(4):608–616.
409. Blumentals WA, Song X. The safety of oseltamivir in patients with influenza: analysis of healthcare claims data from six influenza seasons. *Medscape General Medicine*, 2007, 9(4):23.

410. Dutkowski R et al. High-dose oseltamivir regimens are well tolerated by healthy adults. In: *49th Interscience Conference on Antimicrobial Agents and Chemotherapy (ICAAC)*. San Francisco, CA, 2009:V-1062.

411. Gums JG, Pelletier EM, Blumentals WA. Oseltamivir and influenza-related complications, hospitalization and healthcare expenditure in healthy adults and children. *Expert Opinion on Pharmacotherapy*, 2008, 9(2):151–161.

412. Kawai N et al. Comparison of the effectiveness of zanamivir and oseltamivir against influenza A/H1N1, A/H3N2, and B. *Clinical Infectious Diseases*, 2009, 48(7):996–997.

413. Kimberlin DW et al. Safety of oseltamivir compared with the adamantanes in children less than 12 months of age. *The Pediatric Infectious Disease Journal*, 2010, 29(3):195–198.

414. Lee N et al. Factors associated with early hospital discharge of adult influenza patients. *Antiviral Therapy* 2007, 12(4):501–508.

415. Liem NT et al. Clinical features of human influenza A (H5N1) infection in Vietnam: 2004-2006. *Clinical Infectious Diseases*, 2009, 48(12):1639–1646.

416. Tanaka T et al. Safety of neuraminidase inhibitors against novel influenza A (H1N1) in pregnant and breastfeeding women. *Canadian Medical Association Journal*, 2009, 181(1–2):55–58.

417. McGeer A et al. Antiviral therapy and outcomes of influenza requiring hospitalization in Ontario, Canada. *Clinical Infectious Diseases*, 2007, 45(12):1568–1575.